allergy-free cooking

recipe book

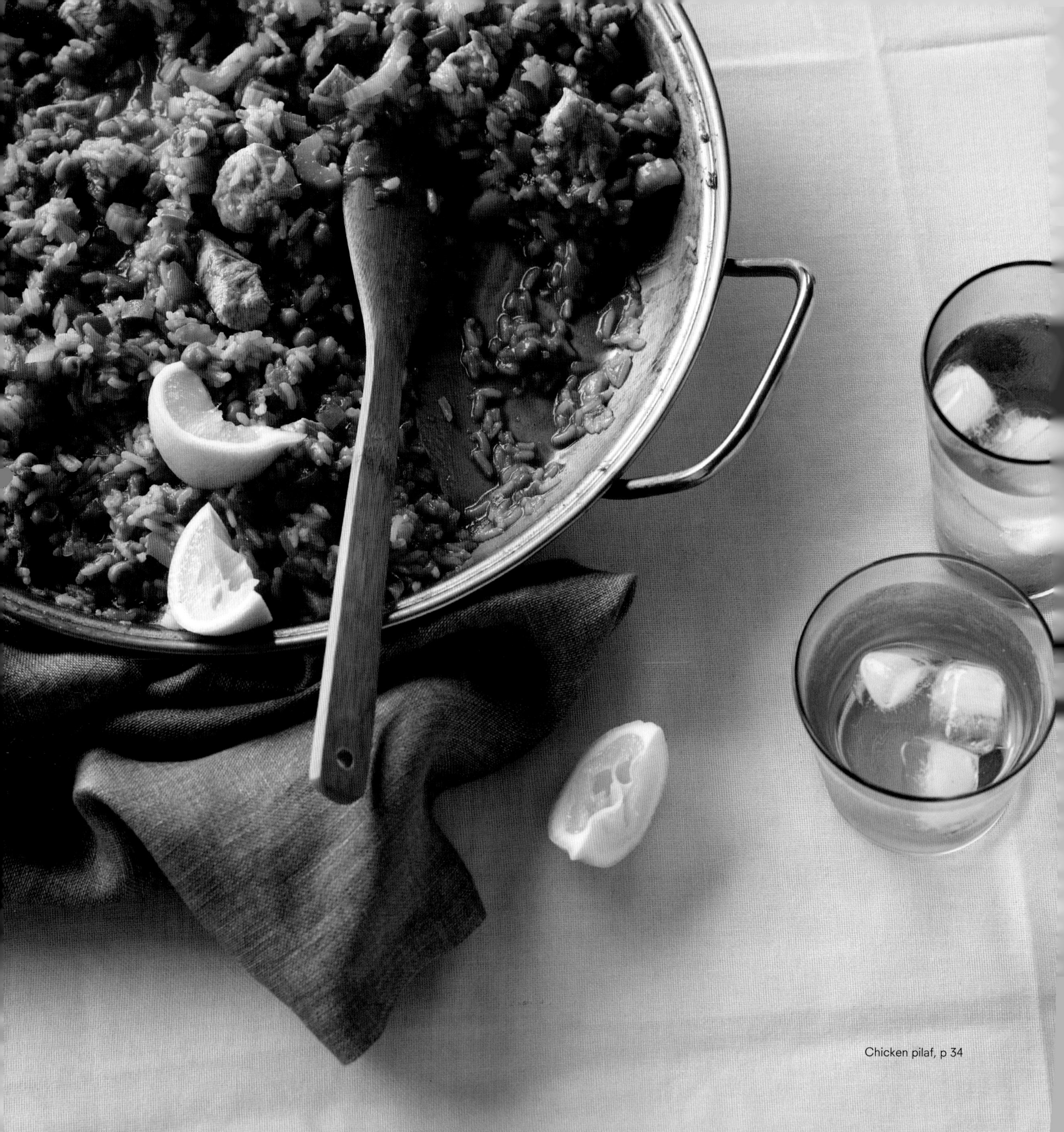

Chicken pilaf, p 34

allergy-free cooking
recipe book

DR SUE SHEPHERD

photography by Rob Palmer

VIKING
an imprint of
PENGUIN BOOKS

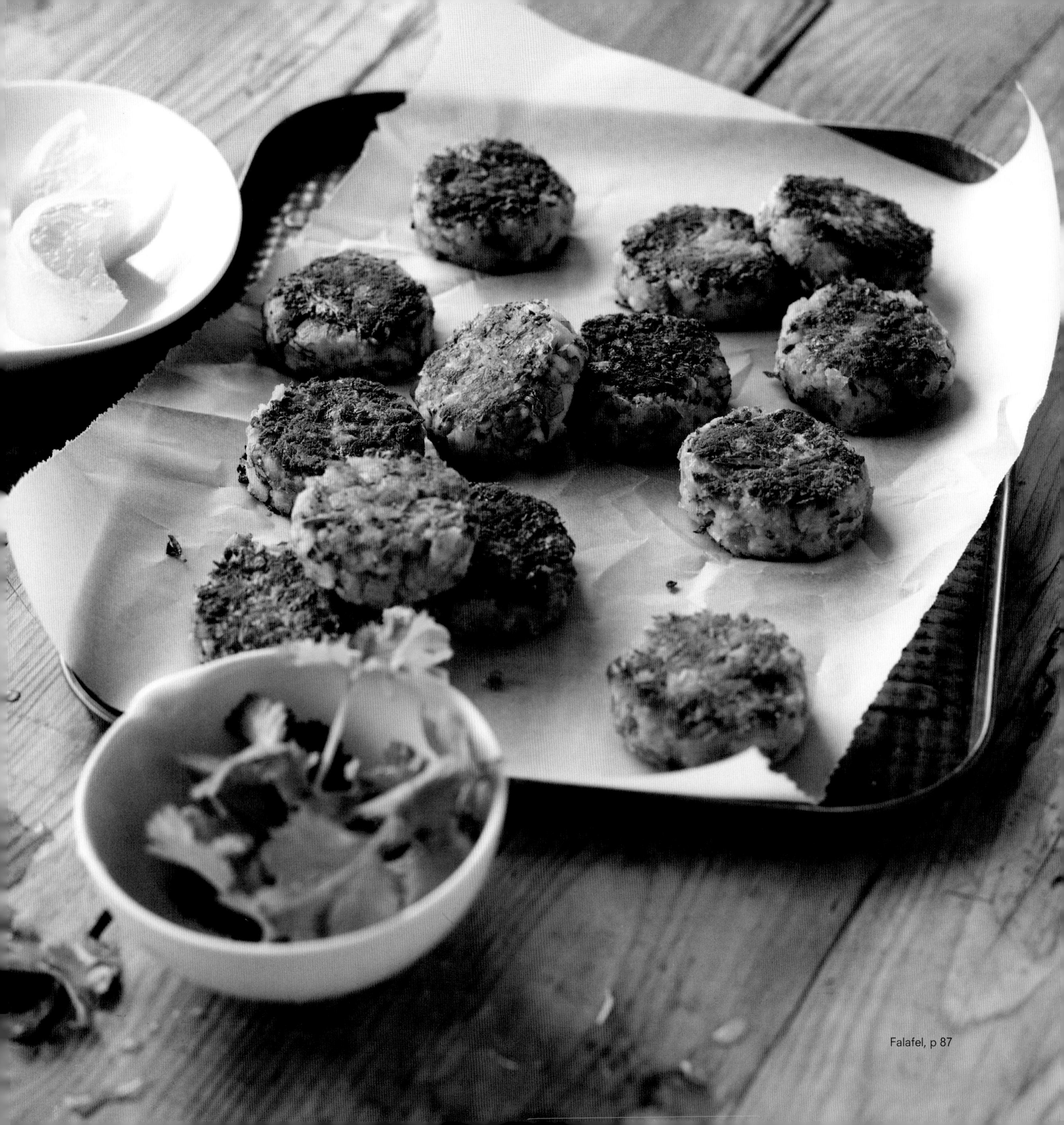

Falafel, p 87

contents

introduction 1
allergy information 2
stocking your kitchen 6

breakfast ideas 13
salads 17
main meals with chicken 31
main meals with meat 49
finger food 81
vegetarian mains 85
meals for kids 103
sweet treats for kids 123
sweets 127
baking 147

acknowledgements 165
index 166

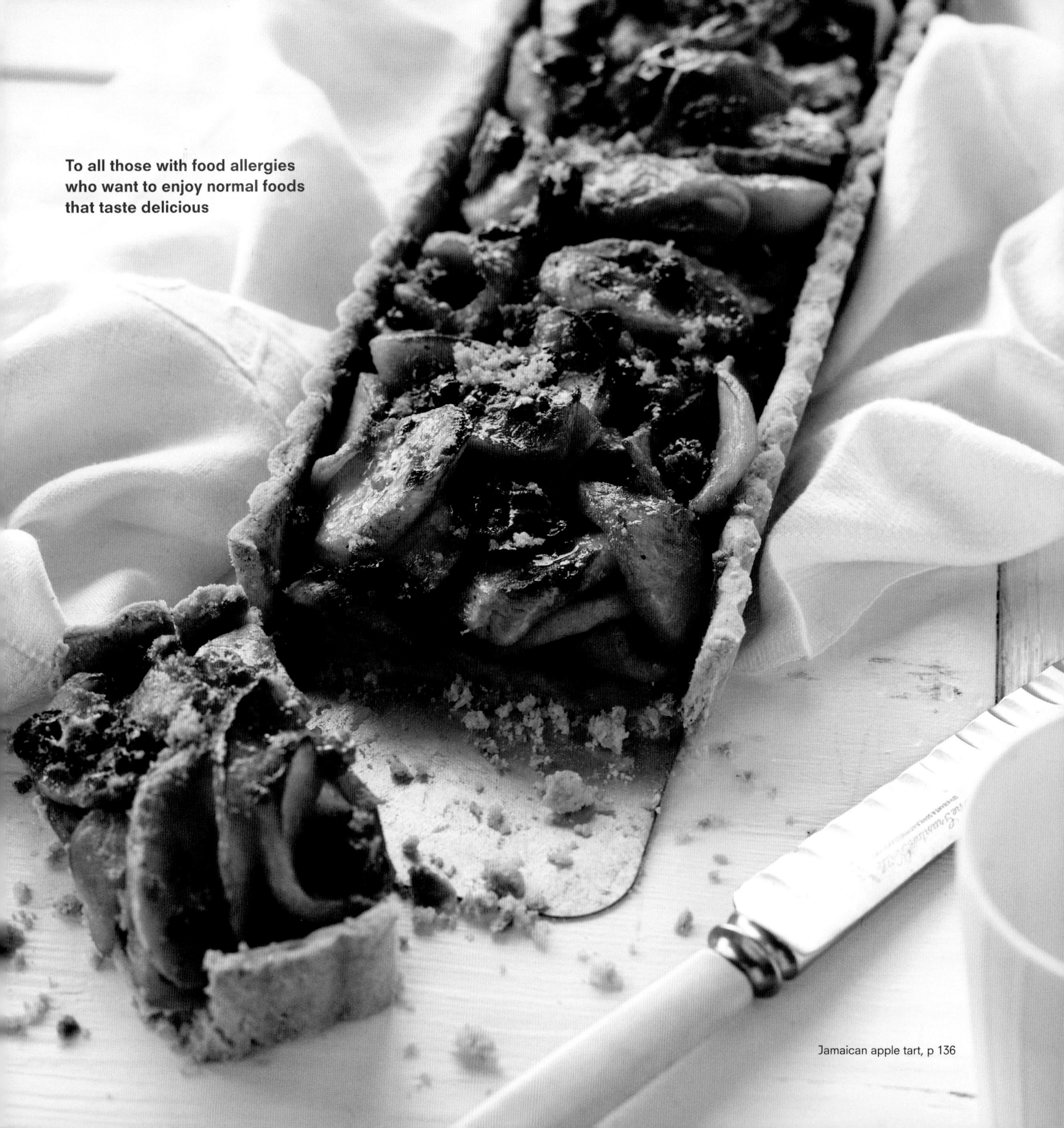

To all those with food allergies who want to enjoy normal foods that taste delicious

Jamaican apple tart, p 136

introduction

If you or someone in your family suffers from food allergies, I'm hoping this unique collection of recipes will be the answer to your prayers. Imagine having the confidence to pick up a cookbook and know you can make everything in it without having to adjust or adapt it to accommodate your allergy. Every recipe on the following pages is free from wheat, gluten, dairy, nuts, seeds, fish and shellfish. Only a very small number of recipes use egg or soy (soy sauce), and if you have an allergy to these, I have provided alternative ingredients and methods for you.

The recipes have been designed with the whole family in mind, so there is no need to cook separate meals – everyone can enjoy them. And I've kept them simple so they are not difficult to make.

I have coeliac disease myself, and know what it is like to live with strict dietary restrictions. In the 16 years since my diagnosis, I have learned that the key to ensuring I don't feel like I am missing out is to maintain an enthusiasm for food, keep my eyes open for new products and enjoy great-tasting safe foods.

In creating this collection of recipes, my main aim is to make lives easier (and tastebuds more contented) for everyone who suffers from food allergies. Happy eating!

– SUE SHEPHERD

allergy information

What is a food allergy?

Food allergies are a type of adverse reaction to food that involve the immune system. In most of us, food is harmless. However, for people who have food allergies, the body has an abnormal immune response to a protein in food. In such instances, the protein is called an allergen. Common allergens include egg, milk, peanuts and tree nuts. Less common are seafood, sesame, soy, fish and wheat.

When people with an allergy eat or drink something containing the allergen, the body's immune system responds by releasing defensive chemicals (including histamine) into the body. These defensive chemicals cause inflammation, and can affect the lung and airways, digestive system, skin and heart/circulatory systems in varying degrees of severity. In food allergy, the specific reaction may be the production of a type of antibody to that allergen or a specific reaction due to other types of immune responses. The type of immunological reaction affects the type of symptoms that result. Symptoms can include mouth irritation (itching, burning, swelling), runny nose, rash on the skin (including hives), nausea and, more seriously, diarrhoea and abdominal cramps/pain, vomiting and difficulty breathing. In severe cases they can be life threatening – a reaction called anaphylaxis.

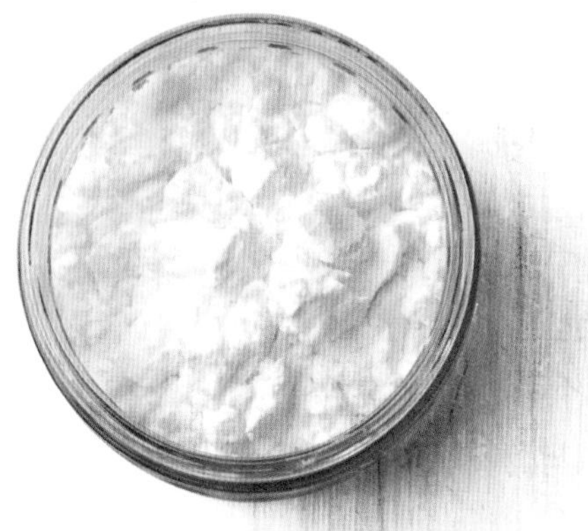

What is the difference between a food allergy, food hypersensitivity and food intolerance?

There are two broad types of adverse reactions to food.

- Food reactions that DO involve the immune system (immunological reaction), as the body reacts to a protein in the food. There are two main types of immunological reactions – food allergy and food hypersensitivity. These are discussed in the next section.
- Food reactions that DO NOT involve the immune system (non-immunological reaction) are referred to as food intolerances. These reactions are more common than immunological reactions. For more information about food intolerance, I suggest you read *Food Intolerance Management Plan* written by myself and Dr Peter Gibson (Penguin Books, 2011).

How do food allergy and food hypersensitivity differ?

Food allergy: In true food allergy, the body makes antibodies known as immunoglobulin E (IgE) to the food protein (the food protein is called an allergen). When the antibodies and the allergen meet up, there is a series of reactions that then occur, resulting in the release of histamine and other defensive chemicals into the body. These chemicals can cause reactions affecting the mouth, gut, skin, lung and airways, and the cardiovascular system. Symptoms can include those described in the 'What is a food allergy?' section, left.

Food hypersensitivity: involves the immune system; however, it does not involve making IgE antibodies. Food hypersensitivity reactions are not as easy to diagnose as allergies as there is not a specific IgE to that protein. In some people, other antibodies (non IgE) have been detected to specific food proteins. Diagnosing food hypersensitivity requires an elimination diet followed by re-challenges with the food components that are queried triggers. This step-by-step method of diagnosing requires great expertise. It is recommended that you seek advice and guidance from doctors and dietitians with experience in food hypersensitivities. Food hypersensitivity may be a trigger in irritable bowel syndrome (IBS) in some people, however IBS is more likely to be triggered by poorly absorbed sugars called FODMAPs – see the book *Food Intolerance Management Plan* for further information.

A special note about coeliac disease

Coeliac disease is a food hypersensitivity that occurs due to an immunological reaction to gluten. Gluten is in the protein component of wheat, rye, oats, barley and triticale. People with coeliac disease can often experience symptoms of IBS, therefore it is essential that all people diagnosed with IBS should talk to their doctor to be investigated for coeliac disease. When coeliac disease is confirmed (diagnosed), then a life-long strict gluten-free diet is followed, in order to reverse the damage to the lining of the small intestine that is caused by the immune reaction to gluten. Unlike other food hypersensitivities, there are very good screening tests (gene tests and blood tests) and excellent diagnostic tests (small bowel biopsy) for coeliac disease.

How common are food allergies?

Prevalence of food allergies is increasing, and is currently estimated to be five times more common in children than in adults. In Australia, approximately one in 20 children have food allergies, compared with one in 100 adults. This suggests that most food allergies will resolve over time; however, peanuts, tree nuts, seeds and seafood are the major food triggers for allergies that last for life.

How are food allergies diagnosed?

It is most important to seek advice from a medical practitioner who specialises in food allergies, such as an Allergist or Clinical Immunologist. Symptoms can vary in type, severity and how quickly they appear.

There may be times when an allergen causes symptoms and other times when it doesn't – this may be due to a threshold of how much allergen can be tolerated before symptoms appear. It is important not to make a diagnosis yourself as you may be incorrect in several ways:

- the reaction may be a food hypersensitivity or intolerance instead
- you may identify the wrong allergen
- there may be multiple allergens
- the reaction may not be due to food but medications, insect bites or other environmental triggers.

A few important points about allergy testing

- Your doctor will likely conduct a series of tests, including a skin-prick allergy test, or blood tests for IgE antibodies to specific allergens (called a RAST test).
- Although allergy testing can provide information about whether a person is allergic, the tests do not reliably predict whether the reaction will be mild or severe.
- A positive RAST indicates that the body's immune system has produced an immunological response to a food. Not all positive results mean there will be a problem reaction. Some people can have a positive result but still eat the food (this is called a false positive result).
- As false positives are possible, your doctor may suggest you confirm the suspected allergen with a doctor/dietitian-supervised food challenge.

An elimination diet removing suspected food allergens should be under the supervision of your doctor and dietitian, followed by rechallenges (reintroduction of specific foods) in order to monitor your response and assist in identifying the cause. These diets are used as a temporary investigation tool – long-term restrictive diets carried out without consultation with a doctor or dietitian are not recommended as they can be nutritionally inadequate.

Which tests are NOT recommended by the allergy medical professionals for food allergy testing?

The Australasian Society of Clinical Immunology and Allergy (ASCIA) is the peak professional body of clinical immunology and allergy in Australia and New Zealand. ASCIA advises that there are many so-called food allergy tests available that may be promoted by many non-medical practitioners. It is important to note that many have no scientific basis and are not useful to diagnose food allergy, or to assist in guiding medical treatment. Please go to the ASCIA website www.allergy.org.au to understand the tests and investigations that are not recommended by the allergy medical experts. Importantly, it also lists the tests and investigations that are scientifically valid.

People with concerns about food allergies are encouraged to obtain information and advice from recognised authorities, including Allergy Centres at major hospitals and also the ASCIA website: www.allergy.org.au.

Can food allergies disappear?

When an allergy develops in adulthood, it is likely that it will be life-long. In children, however, how long a food allergy continues varies considerably from child to child. Typically, children with allergies to soy, wheat, eggs and cow's milk are able to tolerate these by the time they commence school. However, for children with allergies to peanuts, tree nuts, seeds and seafood, these tend to persist into adulthood in the majority (approximately 75%).

How are food allergies treated?

People with food allergies have different management plans, based on how severe the symptoms of the reaction are. All people with food allergies are advised to be treated by a qualified medical practitioner (Allergist or Clinical Immunologist), together with a specialist Accredited Practising Dietitian and other supportive health professionals. These professionals can teach you ways to minimise your risk of eating food allergens. See contacts on page 11. The information that follows describes how to identify allergens in food.

Reading food labels – mandatory declaration of allergens on ingredients lists

It is important to read the ingredients list on food packaging to establish if a food is suitably free of allergens. However, there is a lot of other information on packaging that is useful for you to know.

Understanding information on food labels

Food Standards Australia New Zealand (FSANZ) is the authority that sets food standards covering content and labelling of food sold in both Australia and New Zealand. These standards also apply to food imported for sale in Australia and New Zealand.

FSANZ's main goal is to promote a safe food supply and help consumers to make well-informed decisions regarding their food purchases. Food companies and retailers must comply with food standards (regulations) in the FSANZ Code. These are legal requirements and if they are not followed can result in penalties. For further information on general labelling requirements, visit the FSANZ website www.foodstandards.gov.au.

Requirements for ingredients lists

- Ingredients must be stated in descending order by ingoing weight; that is, the ingredient that is added in its manufacture in the greatest amount is listed first. Water will be listed in order of ingoing weight.
- Very small packets (less than 10 cm × 10 cm) and alcoholic beverages are exempt from listing ingredients, but the supplier must be able to provide this information if requested.
- Imported packaged foods must comply with Australia's food labelling laws. If the original packaging does not comply, a sticker (or similar) will be placed on the food product with the compliant information.
- A law exists for packaged food for the mandatory declaration of ingredients that are derived from a list of defined *allergens*. The list has been formed from those known to cause severe allergic reactions in people (anaphylactic reactions). The following allergens must be declared, no matter how small the amount, if present in packaged food:
  - gluten-containing grains (wheat, rye, barley, oats, and hybridised strains)
  - soybeans and their products
  - milk and milk products
  - egg and egg products
  - fish and fish products
  - crustacea (shellfish) and their products
  - tree nuts and their products
  - peanuts and their products
  - sesame seeds and their products
- Foods that contain sulphite preservatives must be labelled as 'contains sulphites' if they have 10 mg per kilogram or more of added sulphites. It has been set at this level to prevent asthma attacks in susceptible people.
- Additionally, royal jelly (a product made from bees) must be listed with a warning statement, to alert people to the severe allergic reaction that can happen in people with asthma and in those with allergies.
- Processing aids (for example, flour used to dust moulds of confectionery) are declared on the label.
- Compound ingredients are ingredients within the whole food product that have their own ingredients. Take, for example, 'mayonnaise' as an ingredient in a dip. The mayonnaise has its own ingredients. If the compound ingredient (mayonnaise) makes up 5% or more of the final product (dip), all of the ingredients of the mayonnaise will be written (within brackets) within the list of the whole dip's ingredients:

  Spinach dip: Spinach (58%), Mayonnaise (oil, egg, vinegar, salt), Garlic, Salt

  If a compound ingredient (for example, soy sauce powder) makes up less than 5% or more of the final product (such as in a rice cracker), then only allergens present in the compound ingredient will be written (within brackets) within the list of the whole rice cracker's ingredients:

  Teriyaki rice crackers: Rice (85%), Soy Sauce Powder (wheat), Oil, Salt

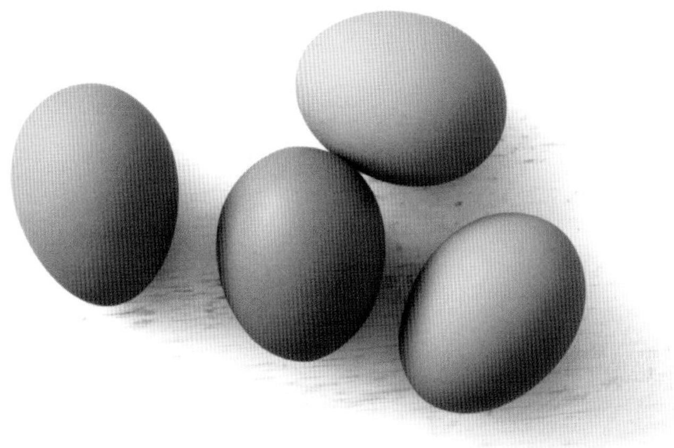

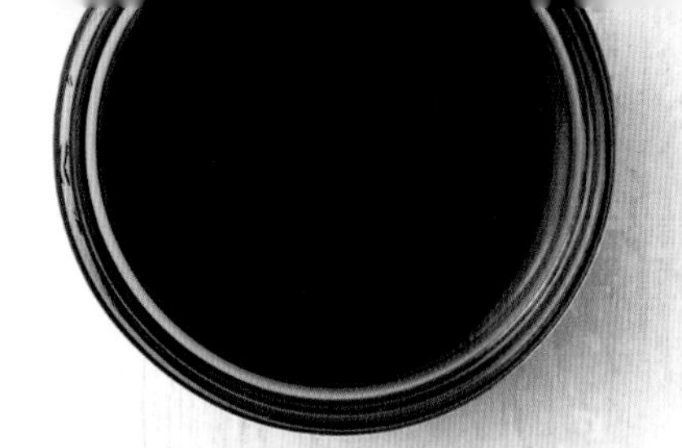

stocking your kitchen

For the sake of convenience, it is a good idea to stock your pantry with the following ingredients. As some ingredients may require a trip to a specialty store, purchase more than you need so you have a good supply on hand.

Flours – alternatives to wheat and soy

Essential:

Cornflour (cornstarch) – must be made from maize (corn); use to thicken sauces, in batters and as part of a flour mix for baking; available in supermarkets

Potato flour – very fine white flour that absorbs moisture; use in flour mix for baking; available at Asian grocery stores

Rice flour – preferably fine rice flour; available at Asian grocery stores; also brown rice flour, which is more nutritious than white flour and has a nutty flavour

Besan flour – an alternative to soy; available in health-food shops and Indian grocery stores

Tapioca flour – also called cassava flour; adds elasticity and chewiness; available at Asian grocery stores

Gluten-free flour – plain and self-raising blends now readily available; check no soy or nuts are present

Worthwhile:

Amaranth flour – useful in flatbreads and baking; available in health-food shops

Arrowroot flour – can take the place of cornflour but quite elastic; available in supermarkets

Buckwheat flour – strong flavour, often used in pancakes and soba noodles; available in health-food shops (be aware that some are blends and contain wheat flour)

Millet flour – good in a flour mix; available in health-food shops

Quinoa flour – used in pasta and breakfast cereal flakes; available in health-food shops

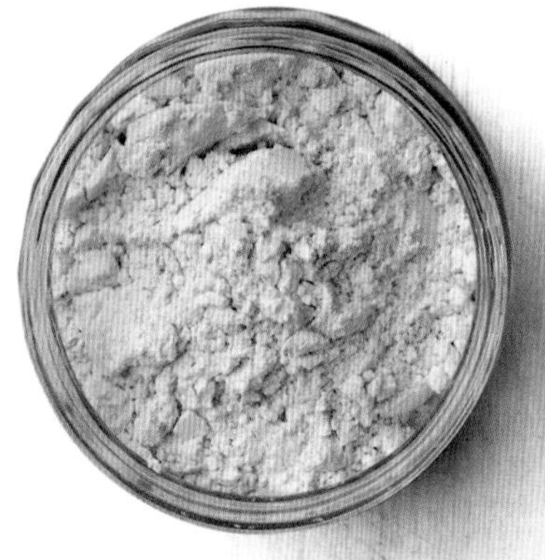

Miscellaneous

Apple cider vinegar (ingredient in a soy sauce alternative)

Balsamic vinegar

Cocoa or carob

Coconut cream (assuming no allergies)

Coconut milk (assuming no allergies)

Dairy-free, soy-free maize tortillas

Dairy-free, soy-free, wheat-free mayonnaise

Dried gluten-free, wheat-free, dairy-free, soy-free breadcrumbs

Egg replacer

Gluten-free baking powder

Gluten-free, wheat-free, dairy-free, egg-free custard powder

Gluten-free, wheat-free, dairy-free, nut-free, soy-free chocolate (dark, milk, white)

Gluten-free, wheat-free, dairy-free, soy-free gravy powder

Gluten-free, wheat-free, dairy-free, soy-free curry powder

Gluten-free, wheat-free, dairy-free, soy-free stock

Gluten-free, wheat-free, dairy-free, soy-free, egg-free pastry sheets

Gluten-free, soy-free, egg-free pasta

Honey

Maple syrup

Molasses (ingredient in a soy sauce alternative)

Mung bean (glass) noodles

Olive oil

Polenta

Popcorn

Psyllium husks (ingredient in an egg replacer)

Rice – brown, white, arborio

Rice milk

Rice paper sheets

Rice vermicelli noodles

Soy-free, dairy-free spread

Sugar – brown, caster, white, pure icing

Xanthan gum (available in health-food shops)

Where to buy specialty allergy-free foods

Many are easy to find these days, but you may have to hunt around for some. The following types of stores are the ones to try.

- **Regular supermarkets and grocery stores:** Most foods are available in major supermarkets and retail food stores. The health-food aisle offers many allergy-free options. The refrigerated and long-life milk sections have milk-free alternatives. Many supermarkets also have Asian sections where you may find some of the wheat-free flours.
- **Health-food stores:** These offer a more extensive range of specialty food than supermarkets, which is increasing in response to greater demand. Obviously, the range differs from store to store, so find one you like and stick to it.
- **Ethnic food stores:** Asian and Indian grocers stock a good selection of wheat-free foods based on rice, tapioca or potato. Prices are usually quite cheap and they often sell foods that are not available in supermarkets or health-food stores.
- **Farmers' markets:** Apart from beautiful fresh produce, these markets often have stalls selling cakes, biscuits, slices and other home-baked goods that are not available through retail stores.
- **Gluten-free retail stores:** These are similar to health-food stores, but all or the majority of items available are gluten-free (wheat-free).
- **Websites and online stores:** These are growing in popularity and number. It's a convenient way to shop and many stores offer an extensive range of allergy-free food options. Purchasing online usually involves courier charges.

The table on the following pages describes the major 'food traps' – foods to be wary of if you have food allergies. It is not exhaustive, so please always check the ingredients of every product you purchase, every time you purchase it.

Common foods that contain allergens

type of allergen | may be found in | The milk and egg rows include their respective products.

breads and cereals

type of allergen	may be found in
milk (products)	high-protein flour
egg (products)	breads
peanuts	breakfast cereals
tree nuts	breakfast cereals, cereals
gluten & wheat	wheat, rye, oat and barley-based foods including pasta, noodles, bread, flatbread, sourdough, breakfast cereals, couscous, semolina, burghal, dry biscuits, breakfast muffins, most gnocchi, kamat, dinkel, spelt flours
sesame seeds	bread rolls and loaves
soy	bread, cereals

meat and meat products

type of allergen	may be found in
milk (products)	deli meats, poultry/turkey (basted), sausages
egg (products)	meatloaf, rissoles/hamburgers
gluten & wheat	corned beef, processed meats, sausages, smallgoods
sesame seeds	pates
soy	bread, cereals

fish and crustaceans

type of allergen	may be found in
fish & shellfish	abalone, calamari, clams, crab, crayfish, cuttlefish, lobster, mussels, octopus, oysters, prawns, scaly or finned fish, shrimps, snails, squid, surimi, yabbies
gluten & wheat	surimi

dairy and dairy-equivalent products

type of allergen	may be found in
milk (products)	butter, buttermilk, casein, caseinate, cheese, cream, creme fraiche, custards and puddings, ghee, margarine with milk products, milk (cow, goat, sheep), milk powder, non-dairy cheeses, non-dairy whiteners, whey
egg (products)	custards, eggnog, egg flips
peanuts	ice-cream
tree nuts	ice-cream
gluten & wheat	soy milks, custards, yoghurts
sesame seeds	bread rolls and loaves

fruit and vegetables

type of allergen	may be found in
peanuts	dried fruit mixes
tree nuts	dried fruit mixes

egg and equivalent products

type of allergen	may be found in
milk (products)	egg replacer

fats and oils

type of allergen	may be found in
milk (products)	margarine spreads
soy	margarine

cuisines

fish & shellfish	most ethnic cuisines
peanuts	African, Asian, Indian, Mexican and vegan dishes
tree nuts	African, Asian, Indian, Mexican and vegan dishes
sesame seeds	Asian and Middle Eastern foods

vegetarian products

gluten & wheat	gluten steaks, textured vegetable protein
soy	bean curd, soybean paste, tofu

mixed meals and snacks

milk (products)	meat pie, soups/soup mixes
fish & shellfish	antipasto, bouillabaisse, caesar salad, pizza toppings (eg anchovy), seafood platters, soups, sushi
egg (products)	frittatas, fritters, glazed foods, omelettes, quiche, souffles, soups
peanuts	health-food bars, salads, snack foods, soup
tree nuts	health-food bars, salads, snack foods
gluten & wheat	breakfast bars, canned soups, flavoured corn chips, flavoured crisps, fritters, frozen dinners, hamburgers, hot chips and wedges, meat pies, muesli bars, packet savoury snacks, pizza, snack foods, souvlaki, stuffed chickens
sesame seeds	nutritional snacks, salads
soy	canned beans, salads

baked goods

milk (products)	baked goods (cakes, etc), pastries
egg (products)	biscuits, cakes (eg sponge, angel), doughnuts, icing on cakes, macaroons, pancakes, pastries, glazed pastries, slices, waffles
peanuts	biscuits, cakes, fillings, pastries
tree nuts	baked goods, biscuits, pastries
gluten & wheat	baked goods (eg breadcrumbs, cakes, croissants, crumpets, doughnuts, muffins), baking mixes, biscuits (sweet, dry), eclairs, pancakes, pikelets
sesame seeds	baked goods, crackers, pretzels

confectionery

milk (products)	caramel lollies, chocolate-coated
egg (products)	confectionery, marzipan
peanuts	chocolates, confectionery, marzipan, nougat, nut brittle, praline
tree nuts	chocolate, confectionery, marzipan, nougat
gluten & wheat	confectionery, licorice, licorice allsorts, many chocolate bars, many filled chocolates
soy	chocolate, carob

desserts

milk (products)	frozen desserts
egg (products)	frozen desserts, meringue, mousse, pancakes, pavlovas, souffle
peanuts	general
tree nuts	frozen desserts
gluten & wheat	cheesecakes, crepes, dairy desserts, dessert pies, ice-cream cones, pastries and flans, profiteroles, tiramisu
sesame seeds	halvah

drinks

milk (products)	flavoured coffees, flavoured drinks, fruit juice
egg (products)	drink mixes, malted drinks
tree nuts	flavoured coffees, flavoured drinks
gluten & wheat	ale, beer, cereal-based coffee substitutes, cereal beverage powders, Guiness, lager, lemon barley cordial, malted milk, soy milk, stout

cooking methods

milk (products)	battered fried foods, canned products
fish & shellfish	fried food in oil used for fish, unclean barbecues
egg (products)	battered fried foods
gluten & wheat	battered fried foods, crumbed foods

sauces and condiments

milk (products)	gravy, salad dressings, sauces and spreads
fish & shellfish	canned spreads, curry pastes, fish sauce, salad dressings, sauces (eg Worcestershire)
egg (products)	salad dressings, sauces (eg Hollandaise)
peanuts	dukkah, gravy, nut spreads/pastes, salad dressings, sauces
tree nuts	chocolate spreads, dukkah, nut pastes/spreads
gluten & wheat	sauces/gravy mixes, soy sauce, stock cubes/powder/liquid, yeast extract spreads
sesame seeds	dressings, marinades, spreads

food additives

milk (products)	flavouring (artificial), flavouring (natural), lactic acid starter culture, seasoned foods
fish & shellfish	cuttlefish ink, flavouring (artificial), flavouring (natural), gelatine, seafood flavouring (eg clam), squid ink
egg (products)	albumen, egg powder, egg white, egg yolk
peanuts	pesto
tree nuts	flavouring (artificial), flavouring (natural), pesto
gluten & wheat	baking mixes/powder, dextrin, flavouring (artificial), flavouring (natural), hydrolysed protein, maltodextrin, starch, textured vegetable protein, thickeners
sesame seeds	dressings, marinades, spreads
soy	emulsifier (322), hydrolysed vegetable protein, lecithin, textured vegetable protein, vegetable gum

other

milk (products)	dips, fat substitutes
egg (products)	dips, fish stock
gluten & wheat	ice-cream cones, icing sugar mixture
sesame seeds	dips
soy	miso, tempeh

Note This list is not complete and should be used as a guide only. Please always check the ingredients of every product you purchase, every time you purchase it.

Allergy-free status of the recipes in this book

When writing this book, my aim was to make the recipes free of all allergens, but it's a simple fact that baked goods taste better with eggs, and stir-fries benefit from a good dash of soy sauce. Because it is highly unlikely that one person will be allergic to all (mandatorily declared) allergens, I have made the recipes cater for all allergens, providing alternatives for those who are unable to eat particular ingredients. This way, everyone can enjoy the recipes.

In short, all the recipes that follow are free from gluten, wheat, dairy, seed, fish, shellfish (crustacea) and peanuts. Some recipes contain small amounts of soy sauce and eggs, but alternatives are provided within the recipe. The majority of recipes are tree-nut free, but a few contain coconut (classified by some as a tree nut). Suggestions regarding coconut are included in the relevent recipes. Please check with your doctor regarding the suitability of coconut in your diet.

The recipes contain some ingredients that may contain sulphites. These include ham, bacon, sausages, soy sauce and dried apricots. If you need to avoid sulphites, please ensure you choose sulphite-free ingredients.

I have attempted to indicate on each ingredient if an allergen is likely to be present, by suggesting you purchase an allergen-free ingredient. However, some unintentional omissions may have occurred. Please check every label every time you purchase a product.

For an updated list of suitable allergen-free ingredients, please go to www.shepherdworks.com.au/shop/category/books and download the pdf document.

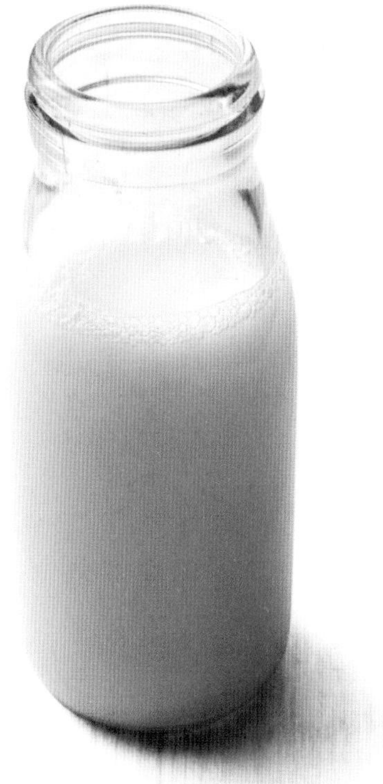

For further information

Australasian Society of Clinical Immunology and Allergy (www.allergy.org.au)

Anaphylaxis Australia, for helpful hints on living with food allergies (www.allergyfacts.org.au)

Dietitians Association of Australia (www.daa.asn.au)

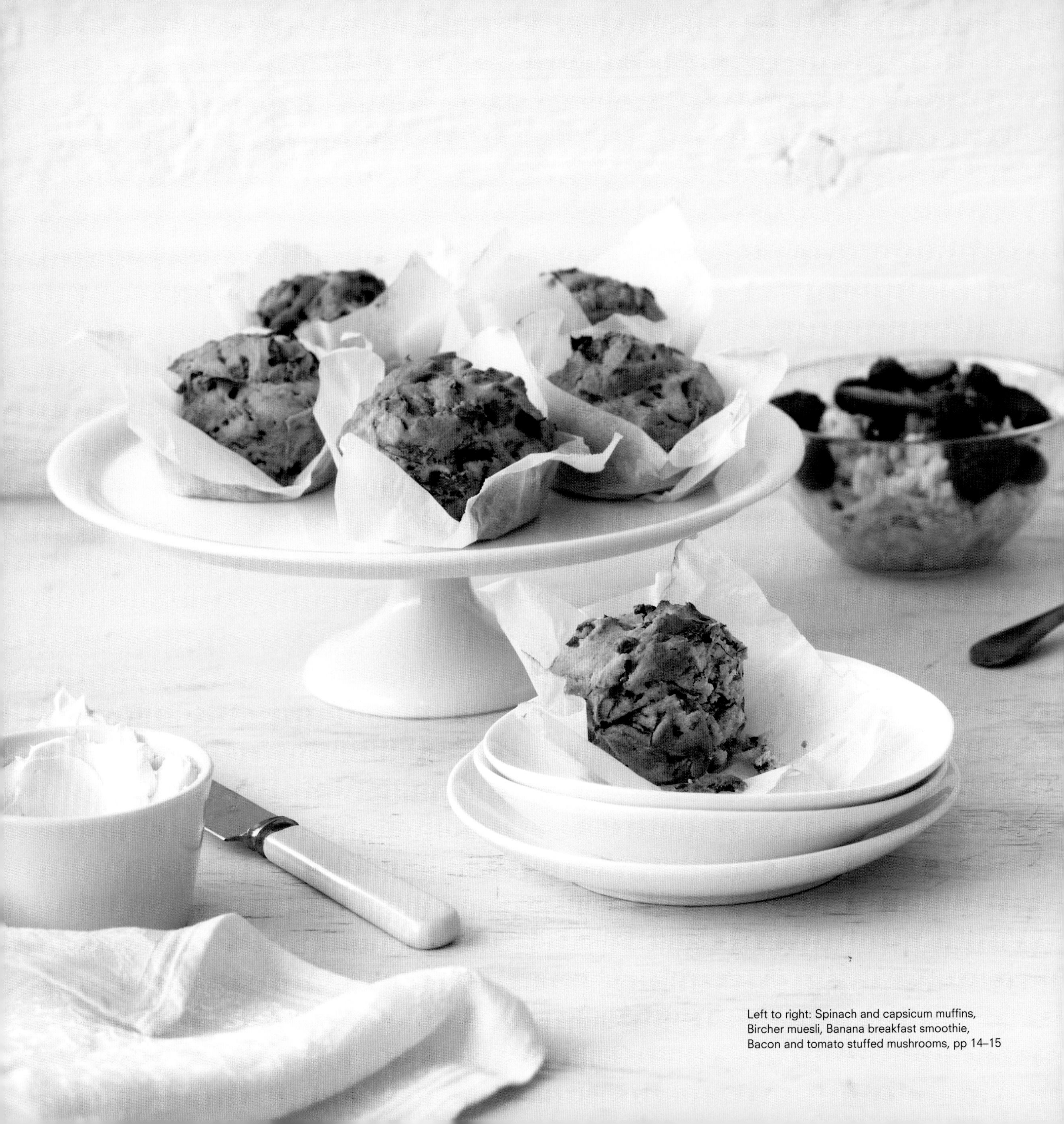

Left to right: Spinach and capsicum muffins, Bircher muesli, Banana breakfast smoothie, Bacon and tomato stuffed mushrooms, pp 14–15

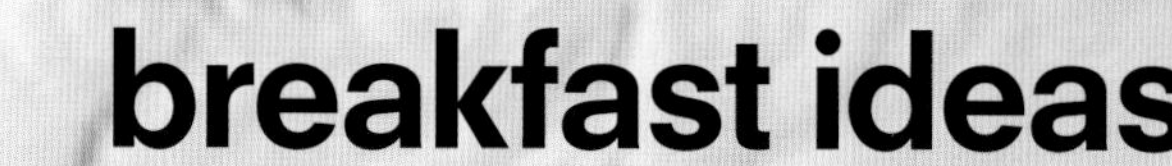

breakfast ideas

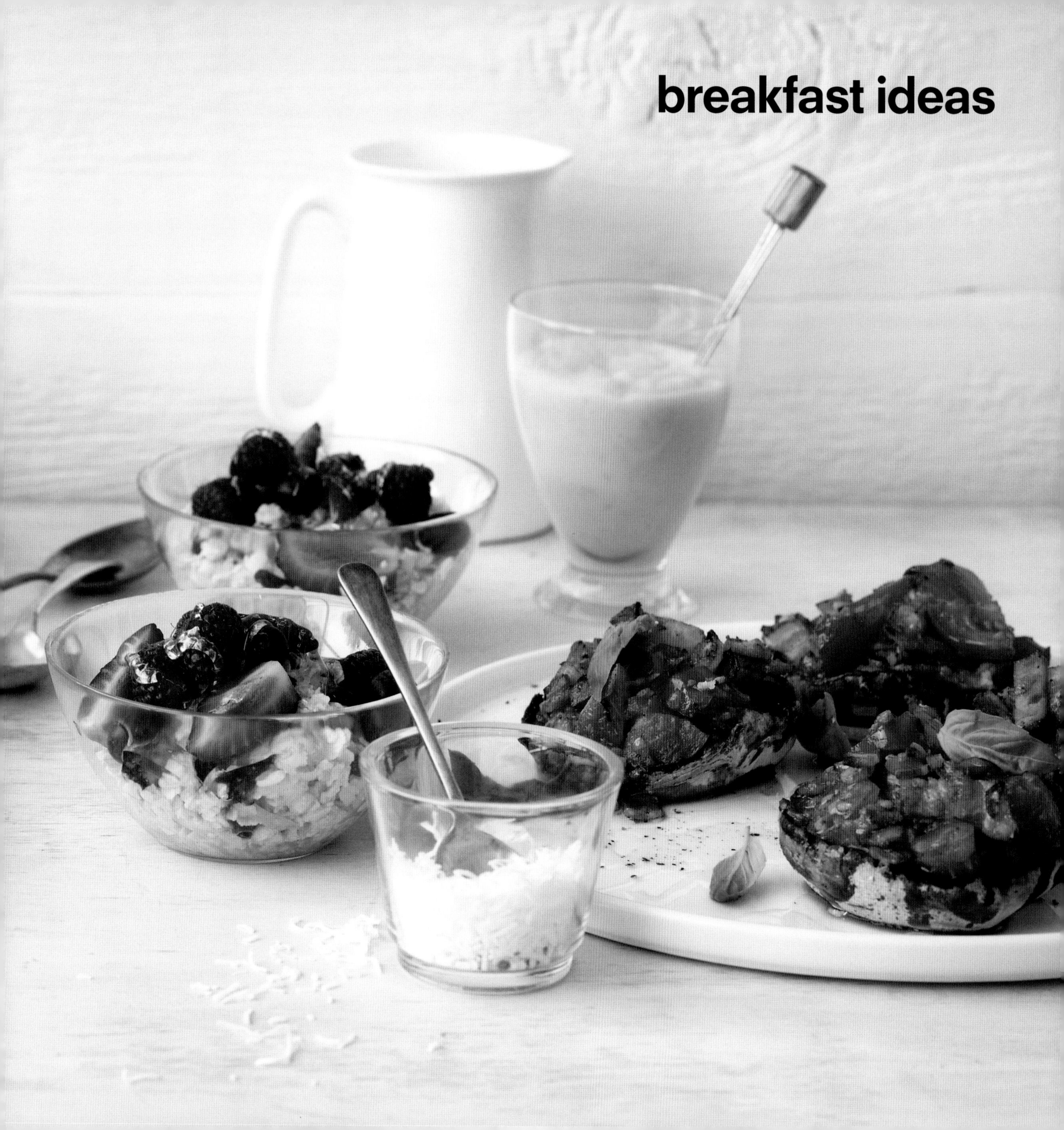

Banana breakfast smoothie

I usually use rice milk in this delicious smoothie, but you could also use oat milk if gluten is not a problem in your diet. Psyllium husks are a great source of soluble fibre and have been included to make the smoothie a bit more 'breakfasty', but they may be left out, if desired.

SERVES 2

2 cups (500 ml) rice milk
2 ripe bananas
4 dried pear halves
1 tablespoon psyllium husks
2 teaspoons honey
6 ice cubes

Place the milk, bananas, pears, psyllium husks and honey in a blender and blend until well combined. Add the ice cubes and pulse until crushed. Pour into two large glasses and serve immediately.

Spinach and capsicum muffins

Fine rice flour is available from Asian grocers, and gives a better texture than the coarser rice flour found in supermarket aisles.

MAKES 12

1 cup (130 g) fine rice flour
½ cup (90 g) potato flour
½ cup (45 g) besan flour
2 teaspoons gluten-free baking powder
1 teaspoon bicarbonate of soda
1 teaspoon xanthan gum
½ teaspoons dried chilli flakes
½ small red capsicum (pepper), seeded and finely diced
80 g soy-free, dairy-free spread, melted
1½ cups (375 ml) rice milk
1 egg, lightly beaten*
100 g baby spinach leaves, shredded
2 tablespoons flat-leaf parsley leaves, finely chopped
1 tablespoon chopped chives
salt and freshly ground black pepper

Preheat the oven to 150°C. Grease a 12-hole muffin tin or line with paper cases.

Sift the flours, baking powder, bicarbonate of soda and xanthan gum into a large mixing bowl and stir through the chilli flakes.

Place the capsicum, dairy-free spread, rice milk, egg, spinach, parsley and chives in a medium bowl. Season to taste with salt and pepper and stir until well combined.

Pour the wet mixture into the dry ingredients and beat with a metal spoon for 2 minutes. Spoon the batter into the muffin holes to about two-thirds full. Bake for 12–15 minutes or until firm to the touch (a skewer inserted into the centre should come out clean). Allow to stand for 5 minutes, then remove from the tin and cool on a wire rack. Serve warm or at room temperature.

***For egg allergy**
Place 2 teaspoons psyllium husks in a small bowl and pour over ½ cup (125 ml) boiling water, stirring constantly to ensure the psyllium does not clump together. Set aside for 4–5 minutes until it forms a gel, stirring occasionally. Use in place of the egg.

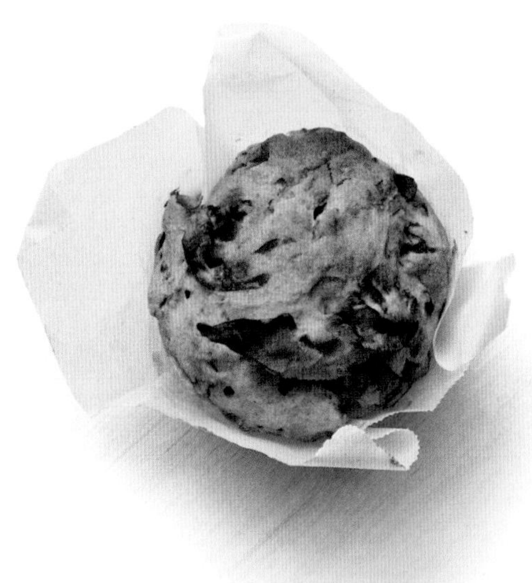

Bacon and tomato stuffed mushrooms

I really enjoy mushrooms at any time of the day. Here, they are served with the traditional breakfast flavours of bacon and tomato, but you can make a vegetarian variation by omitting the bacon. SERVES 4

2 teaspoons olive oil
2 cloves garlic, crushed
1 small onion, finely chopped
2 rashers rindless bacon, finely chopped
3 tomatoes, roughly chopped
4 field mushrooms
3 tablespoons basil leaves

Preheat the oven to 180°C. Line a large baking tray with baking paper.

Heat the olive oil in a small frying pan over medium–high heat and saute the garlic, onion, bacon and tomato for 6–8 minutes or until the tomatoes start to soften.

With a damp cloth, wipe clean the outer skin of the mushrooms. Remove the stems and place the caps on the baking tray.

Fill the caps with the tomato mixture and bake for 7–10 minutes. Remove from the oven and cover with foil for 5 minutes to help the mushrooms soften. Sprinkle the basil leaves over the top and serve warm.

Bircher muesli

Traditional bircher muesli is made using oats. Oats are not gluten free, however they are wheat free (check the label specifies 'wheat-free oats' as many have wheat contamination). This wholesome muesli is so moist and flavoursome it doesn't need the traditional yoghurt accompaniment. If you are allergic to coconut, use rice milk in place of the coconut milk and omit the shredded coconut – it will still taste great! SERVES 4

2 cups (250 g) rolled brown rice flakes
2 tablespoons sultanas
1 cup (250 ml) apple juice
juice of 1 lemon
1 cup (170 g) grated apple
½ cup (125 ml) coconut milk
2 tablespoons honey, plus extra to serve (optional)
1 tablespoon shredded coconut
1 cup (140 g) mixed berries (such as strawberries, blueberries and raspberries)
ground cinnamon, for dusting

Gently combine the rice flakes, sultanas, apple juice, lemon juice, apple, coconut milk and honey in a medium bowl and leave to soak for 1 hour.

Spoon the muesli into four bowls, sprinkle the shredded coconut and berries over the top and drizzle with a little extra honey, if using.

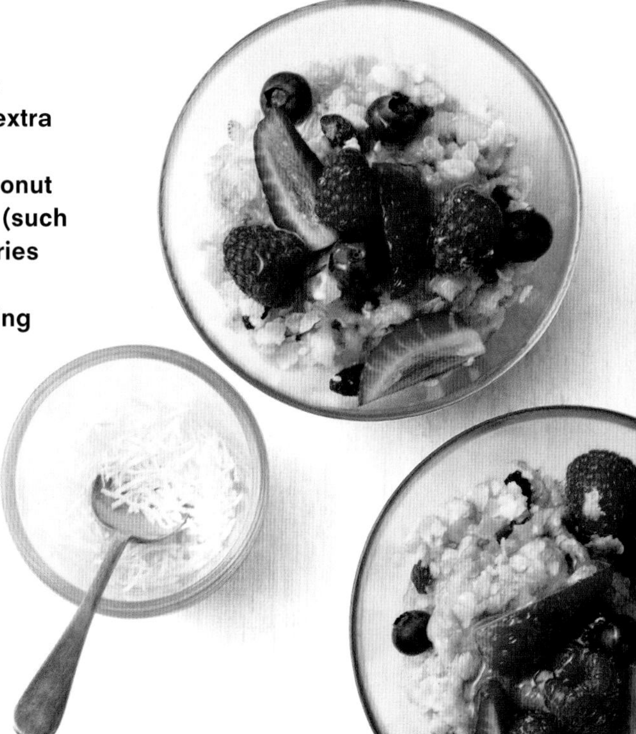

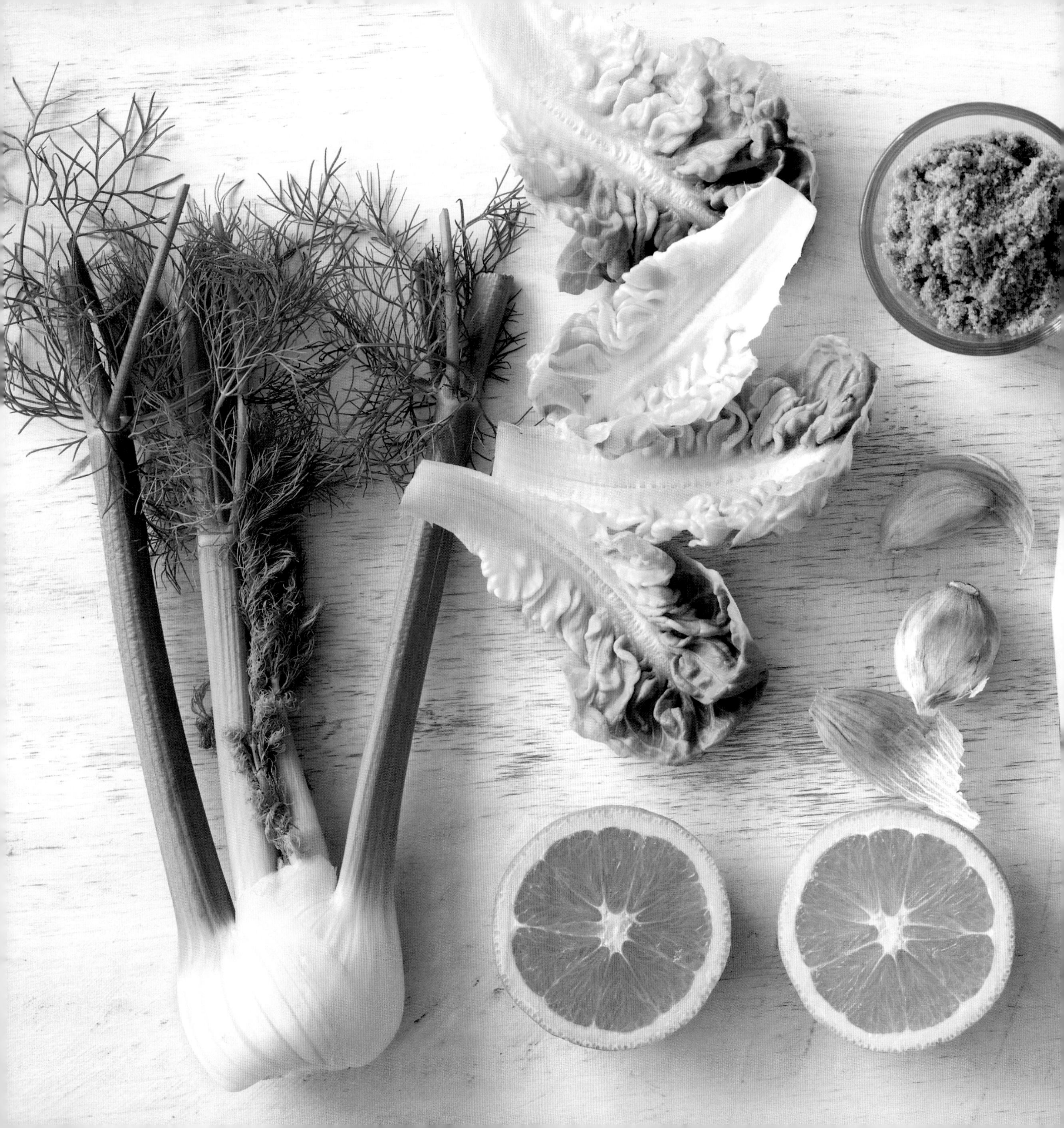

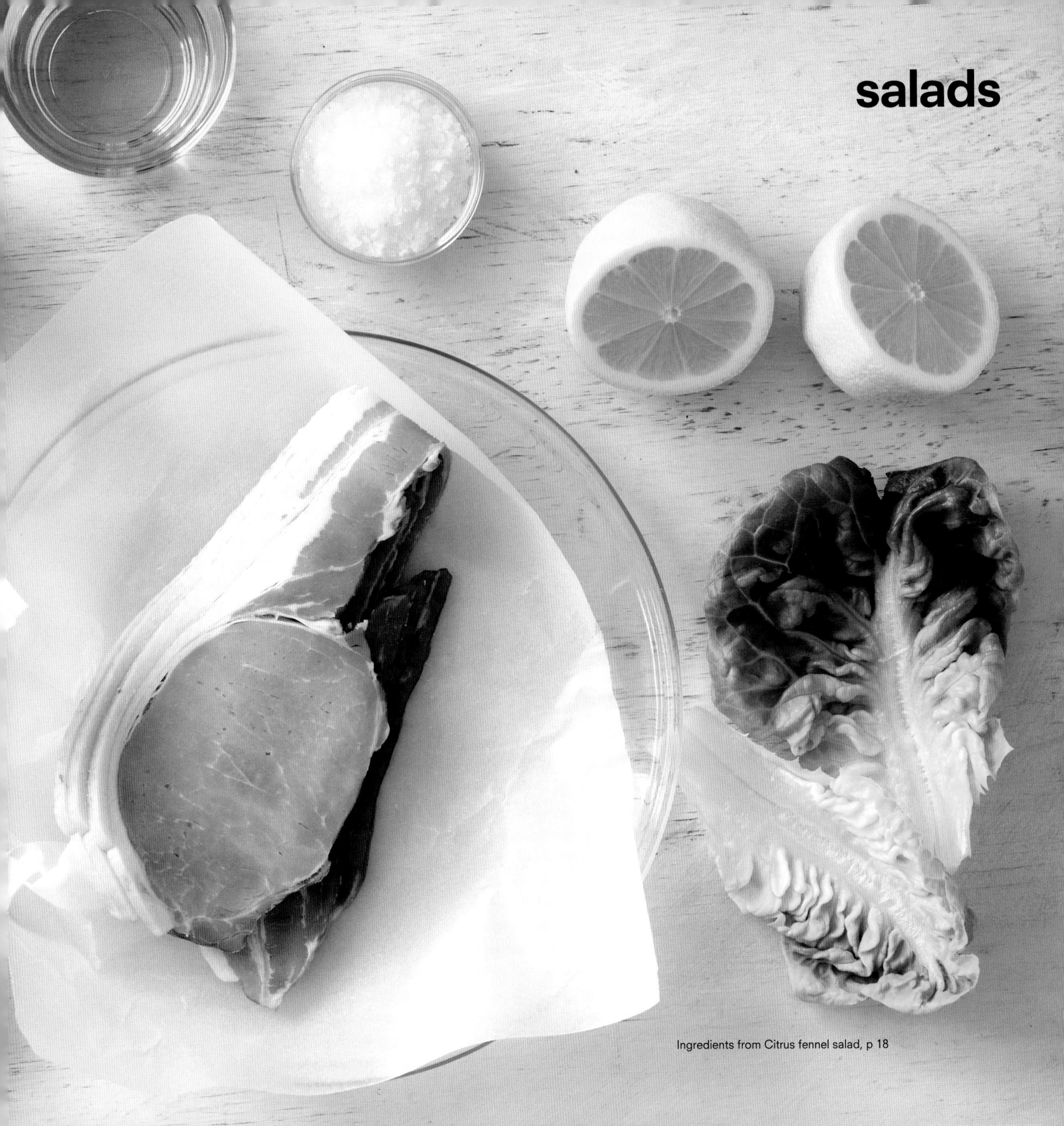

salads

Ingredients from Citrus fennel salad, p 18

Chickpea salad with zucchini and chilli

Chickpeas are a sensational vegetarian source of protein – they have a subtle flavour and mealy texture that may be enjoyed hot or cold. Adjust the quantity of sambal oelek to suit your taste for chilli. SERVES 4

2 × 400 g tins chickpeas, drained and rinsed
3 tablespoons olive oil
2 tablespoons lemon juice
2 teaspoons gluten-free, wheat-free, dairy-free, soy-free Dijon mustard
1 teaspoon sambal oelek (chilli paste)
1 clove garlic, crushed
1 large zucchini (courgette)
3 tomatoes, cut into thin wedges
2 spring onions, green part only, chopped
3 tablespoons chopped chives
3 tablespoons flat-leaf parsley leaves

Combine the chickpeas, olive oil, lemon juice, mustard, sambal oelek and garlic in a bowl. Cover and marinate in the fridge for 3–4 hours.

Use a potato peeler to peel slices down the length of the zucchini. Add to the chickpea mixture, along with the remaining ingredients and toss to combine. Serve at room temperature or cold, if preferred.

Citrus fennel salad >

What I particularly like about this light salad is the range of textures in every mouthful: the crunch of fennel and crisp bacon, complemented by soft baby cos and fresh, juicy orange. SERVES 4

3 rashers rindless bacon, chopped
2 oranges
2 baby bulbs fennel, finely sliced
2 baby cos lettuces, roughly chopped
salt and freshly ground black pepper

DRESSING
3 tablespoons extra virgin olive oil
1 clove garlic, crushed
salt and freshly ground black pepper
3 tablespoons lemon juice
3 teaspoons brown sugar

To make the dressing, place all the ingredients in a small screw-top jar and shake well to combine.

Saute the bacon in a small non-stick frying pan over medium heat until crispy. Remove from the pan and drain on paper towels.

Peel and segment the oranges, then cut into thin wedges.

In a large bowl, mix together the fennel, cos lettuce, bacon and orange wedges. Pour over the dressing and toss well to combine. Season to taste and serve.

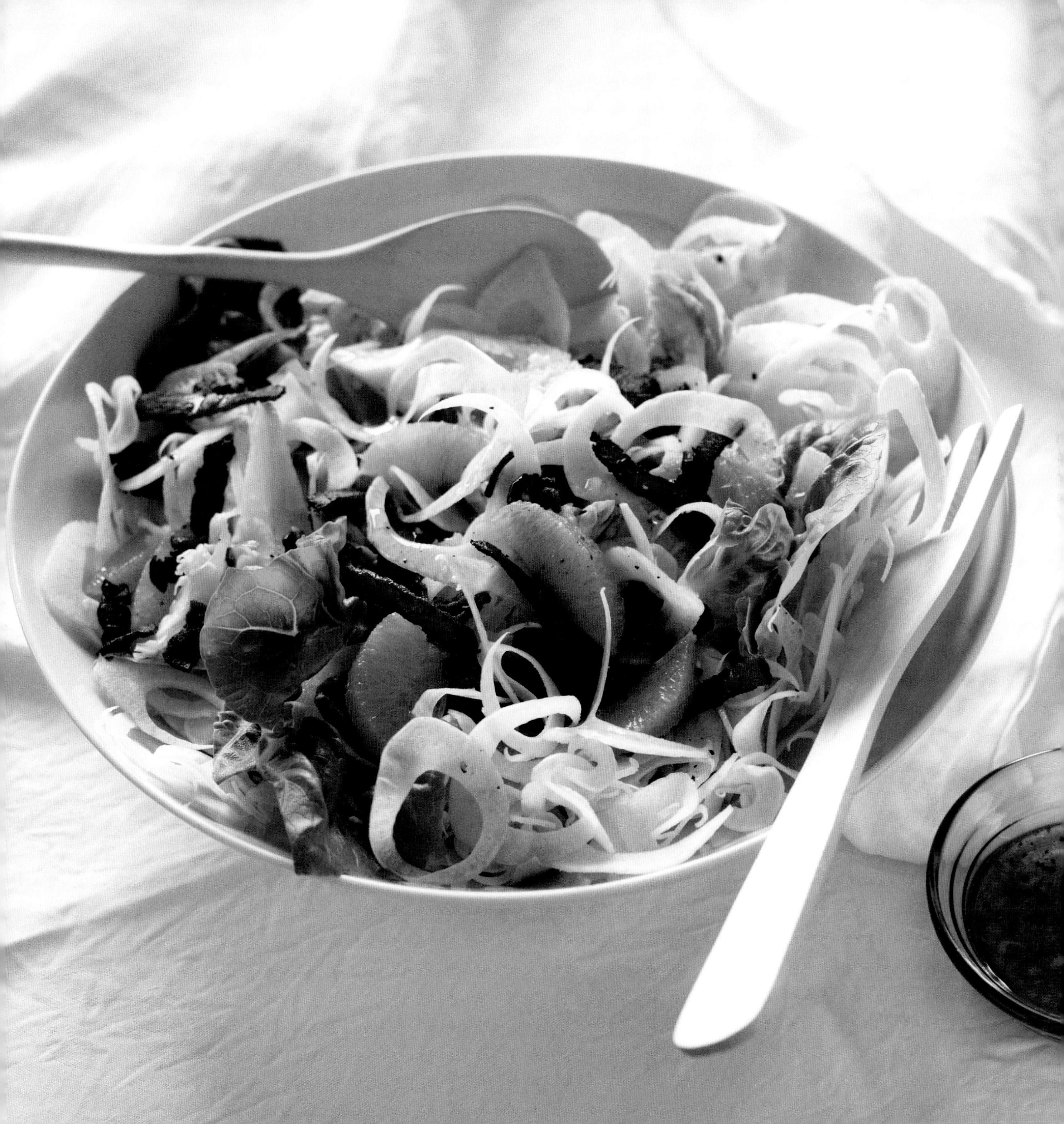

Asian chicken coleslaw

The star of this colourful salad is really the fresh herbs. Adding shredded chicken makes it substantial enough to enjoy on its own, or serve it as an accompaniment.

SERVES 4

2 × 250 g skinless chicken breast fillets
¼ small savoy cabbage, shredded
¼ purple cabbage, shredded
4 carrots, grated
1 cup mint leaves
1 cup coriander leaves

DRESSING
3 tablespoons gluten-free, wheat-free sweet chilli sauce
1 tablespoon lime juice

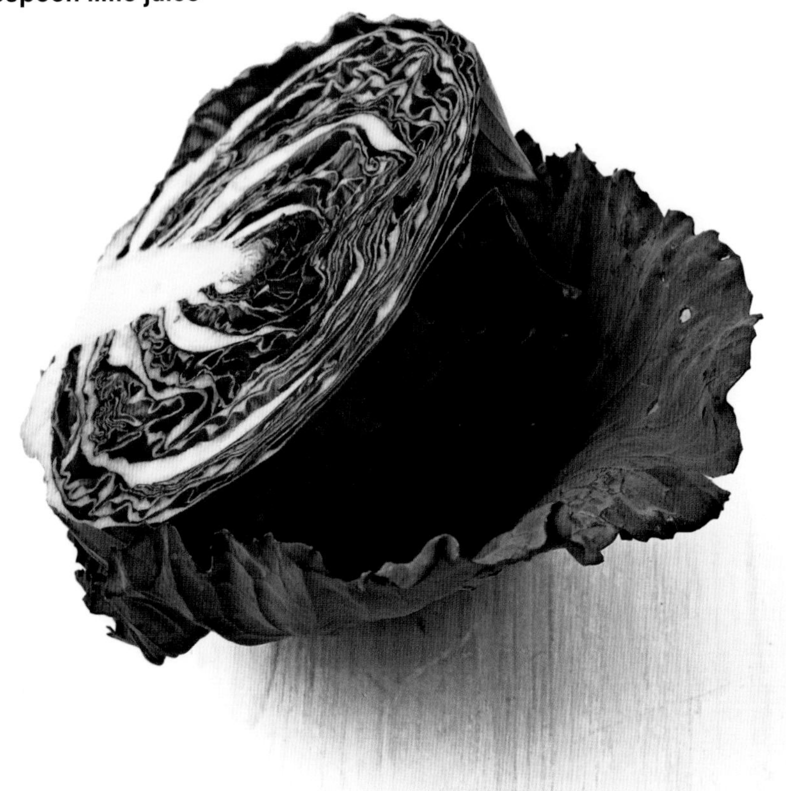

Pour water into a small frying pan or medium saucepan until three-quarters full and bring to the boil. Add the chicken breasts, then reduce the heat to medium and simmer, covered, for 10 minutes or until the chicken is cooked through. Remove from the water and set aside to cool.

To make the dressing, place all the ingredients in a small screw-top jar and shake well to combine.

Shred the cooled chicken breasts with your fingers, then place in a large bowl or platter with the cabbage, carrot, mint and coriander. Drizzle over the dressing and toss gently until combined.

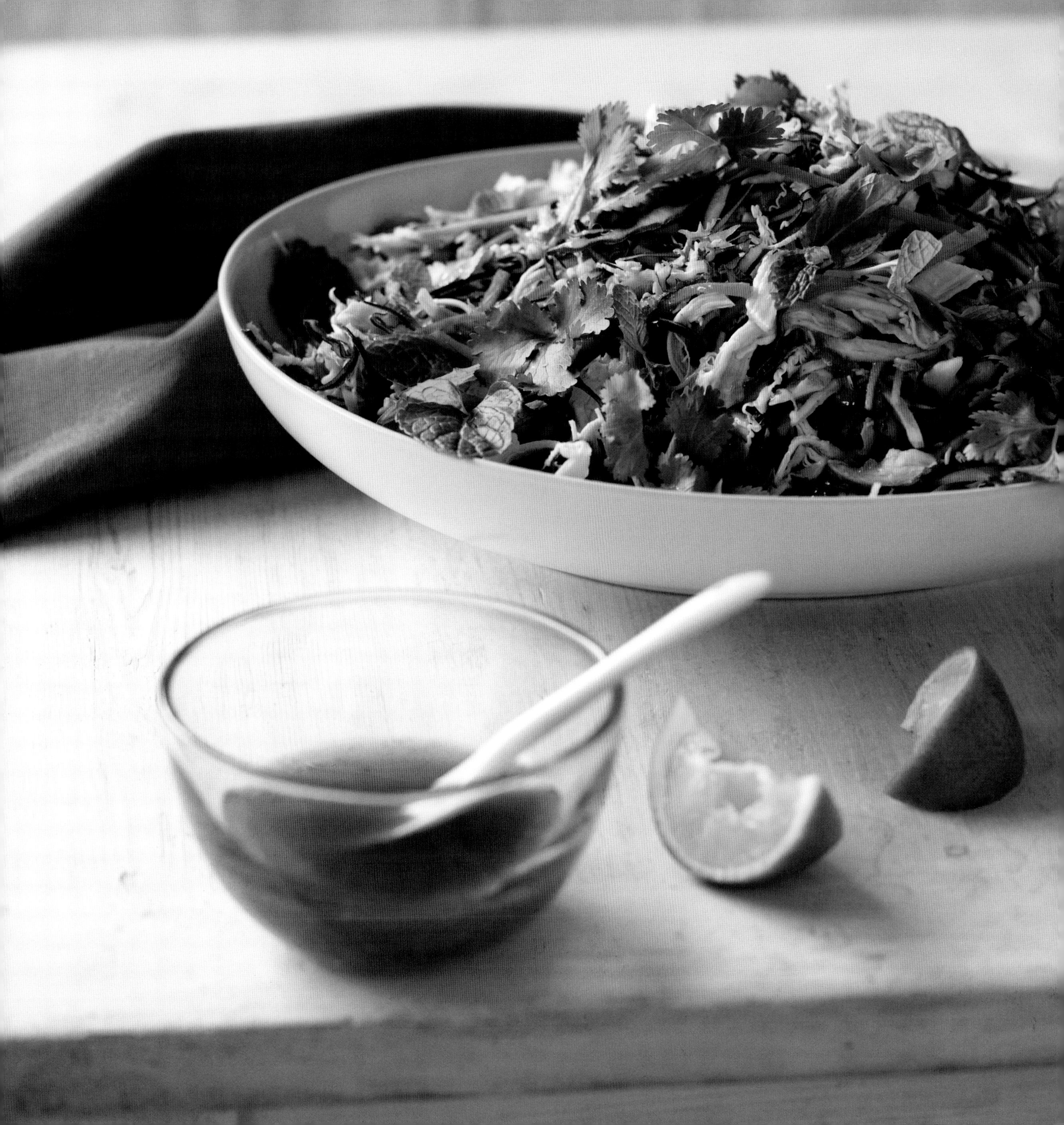

Pear and rocket salad

Rocket and pear is a classic pairing, needing little adornment. As with any simple dish, it is essential to use good-quality ingredients: in this case, fresh, seasonal produce and a fruity extra virgin olive oil. SERVES 2

3 tablespoons extra virgin olive oil
1 tablespoon red-wine vinegar
1 teaspoon gluten-free, wheat-free wholegrain mustard
1 teaspoon honey
1 pear, thinly sliced
3 cups (100 g) baby rocket leaves

Place the olive oil, vinegar, mustard and honey in a small screw-top jar and shake well to combine. Set aside to let the flavours infuse.

Place the pear and rocket in a large salad bowl, add the dressing and toss well to combine.

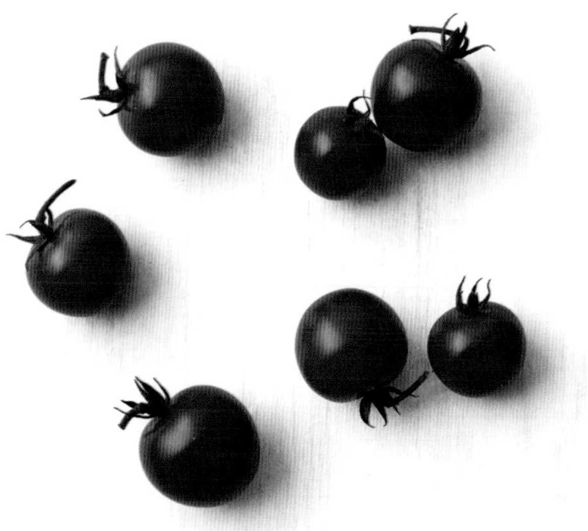

Garden salad with avocado >

Watercress and avocado are two of my favourite salad ingredients, and are perfect in this vibrant salad full of goodness and flavour. SERVES 4

1 cos lettuce, cut into 8 wedges
1 cup (30 g) watercress
1 avocado, cut into large pieces
2 sticks celery, thinly sliced on the diagonal
12 firm cherry tomatoes, cut in half

DRESSING
1 tablespoon gluten-free, wheat-free wholegrain mustard
3 tablespoons extra virgin olive oil
1 tablespoon lemon juice
1 teaspoon grated lemon zest
1 teaspoon balsamic vinegar
1 tablespoon brown sugar

To make the dressing, place all the ingredients in a small screw-top jar and shake well to combine. Set aside to let the flavours infuse.

Combine the lettuce, watercress, avocado, celery and tomato in a large salad bowl. Drizzle the dressing over the top and toss gently to coat.

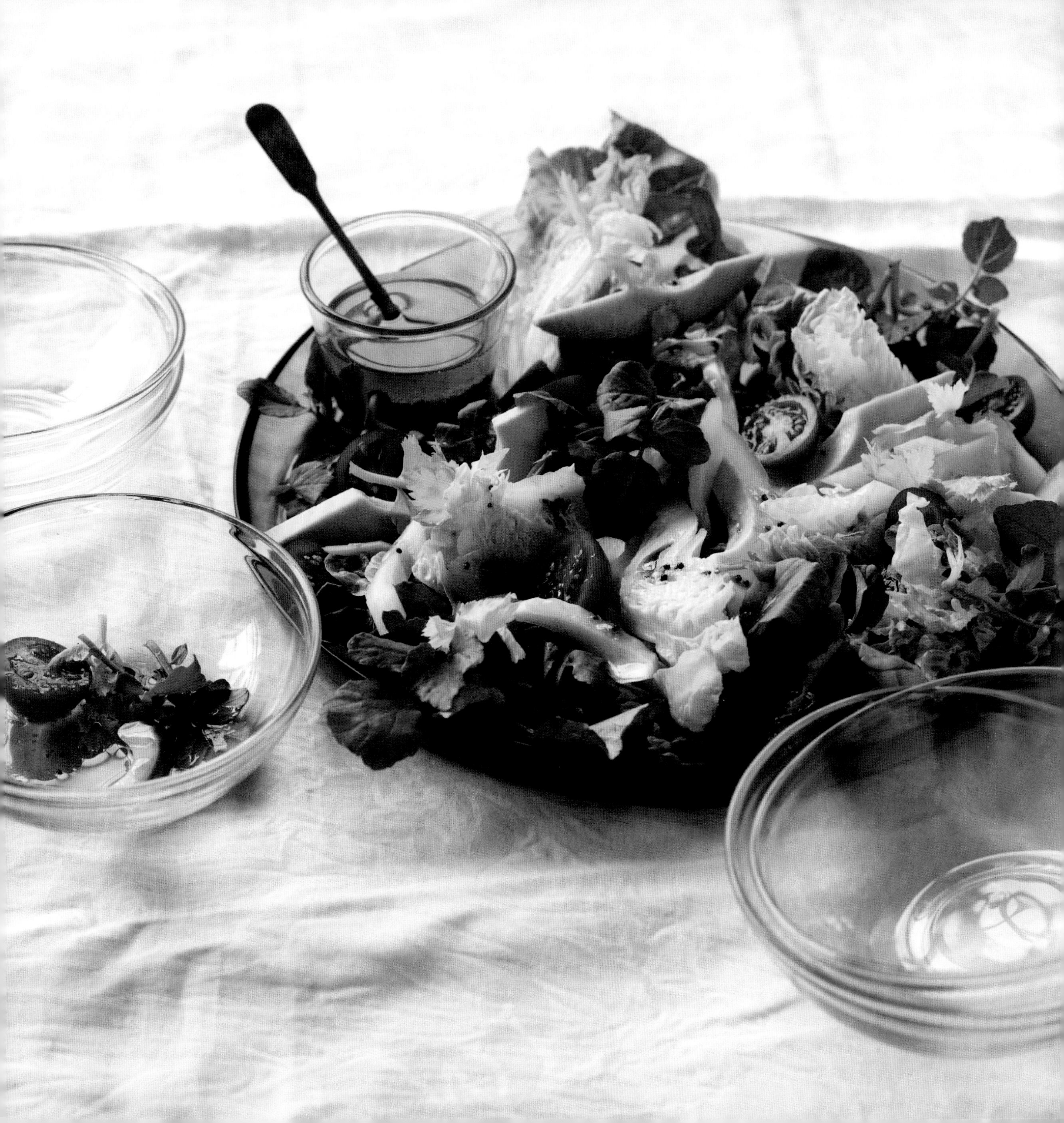

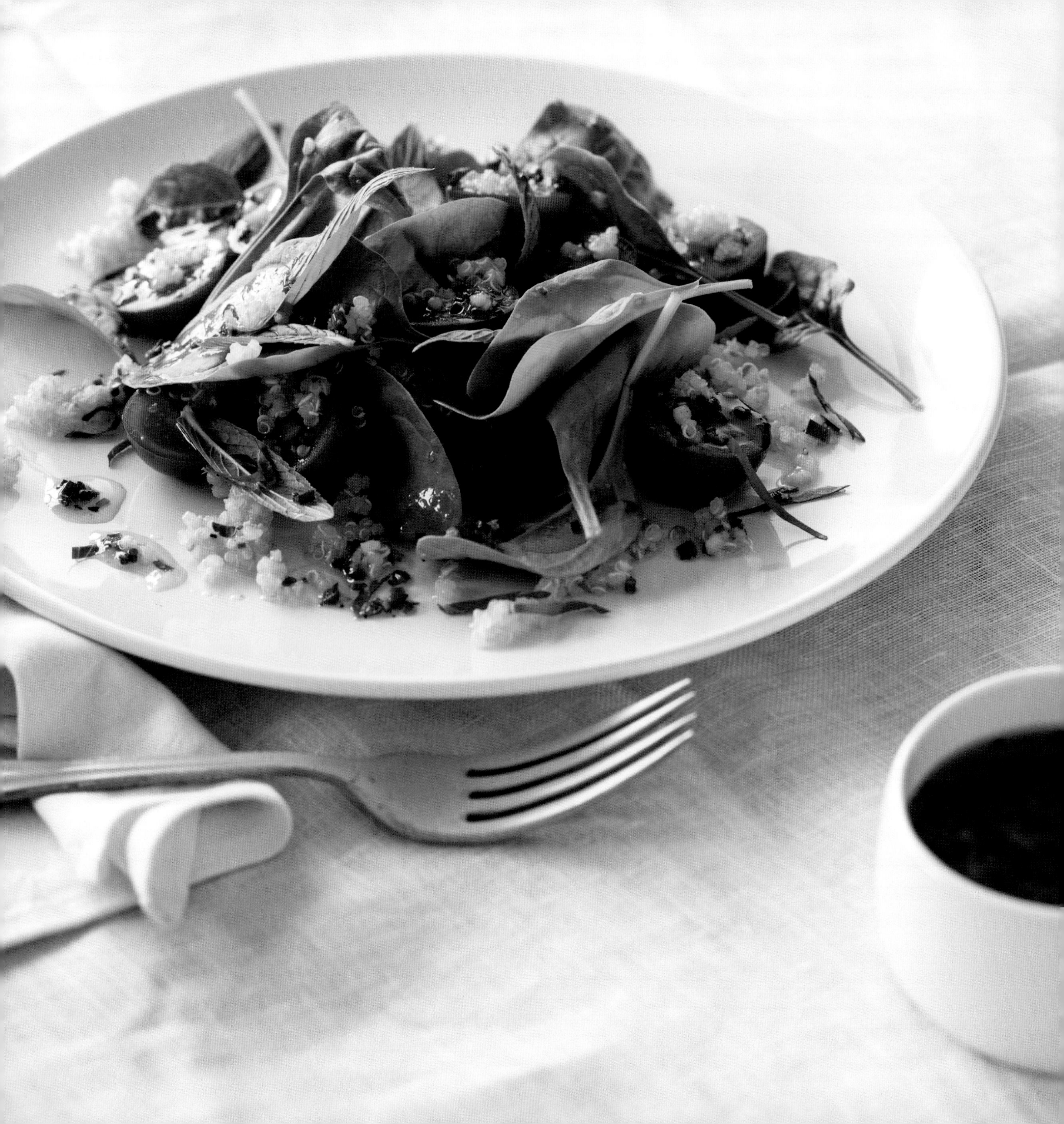

Quinoa salad with mint and lemon

Quinoa (pronounced 'keen-wah') is a new favourite of mine. If you have not tried this nutritious grain before, pick some up at your local health-food shop and welcome it into your recipe repertoire, starting with this zesty salad. SERVES 4

1 cup (100 g) dried quinoa, rinsed and drained
12 cherry tomatoes, halved
2 cups (60 g) baby spinach leaves
2 tablespoons roughly chopped mint

DRESSING
3 tablespoons extra virgin olive oil
1 tablespoon lemon juice
1 teaspoon grated lemon zest
1 clove garlic, crushed
½ teaspoon finely chopped red chilli
1 tablespoon finely chopped flat-leaf parsley
2 tablespoons chopped chives

Pour 1 litre water into a small saucepan and bring to the boil. Reduce the heat to medium, add the quinoa and cook, stirring regularly, for 12–15 minutes or until the quinoa is tender and all the water has been absorbed. Set aside to cool to room temperature.

To make the dressing, place all the ingredients in a small screw-top jar and shake well to combine.

Place the quinoa, tomato, spinach, mint and dressing in a large bowl and toss gently to combine. Cover and refrigerate for 20–30 minutes to allow the flavours to infuse before serving.

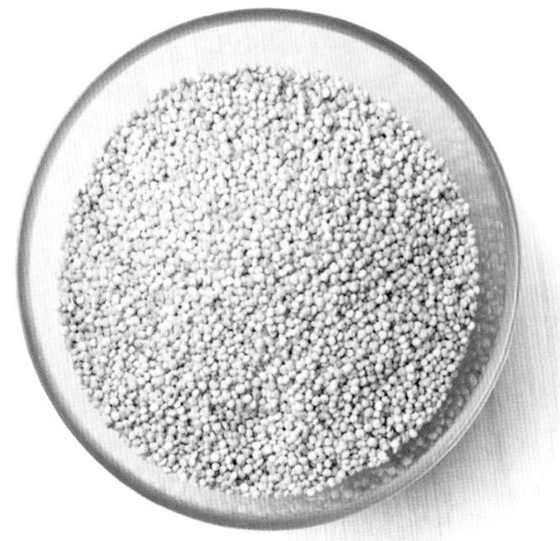

Sweet potato, prosciutto and green bean salad

This is a colourful twist on traditional potato salad – fresh green beans, vibrant orange sweet potato and the salty hit of crisp prosciutto. SERVES 4

500 g orange sweet potato, peeled and cut into 3 cm cubes
olive oil, for drizzling
75 g prosciutto
500 g cocktail kipfler potatoes, cut in half
200 g green beans, trimmed
3 tablespoons gluten-free, wheat-free, dairy-free, soy-free mayonnaise*
salt and freshly ground black pepper

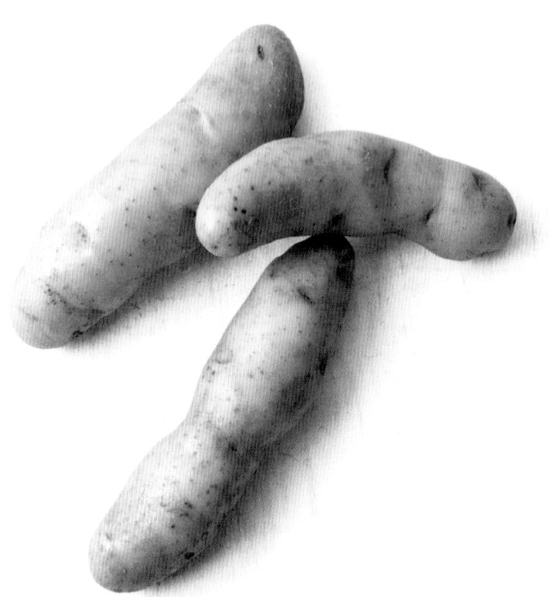

Preheat the oven to 180°C.

Place the sweet potato on a baking tray, drizzle with a little olive oil and bake for 40 minutes or until golden brown, turning occasionally. Set aside to cool.

Meanwhile, place the prosciutto on another baking tray and bake for 15 minutes or until crisp. Set aside to cool.

Cook the kipfler potato in a medium saucepan of boiling water until just tender. Drain and transfer to a large heatproof bowl.

Cook the beans in a small saucepan of boiling water until just tender. Drain and add to the potato.

Break the crisp prosciutto into small pieces and add to the potato and beans, along with the sweet potato. Add the mayonnaise and stir until the vegetables are well coated. Season to taste, then cool in the fridge before serving.

***For egg allergy**
Use egg-free mayonnaise.

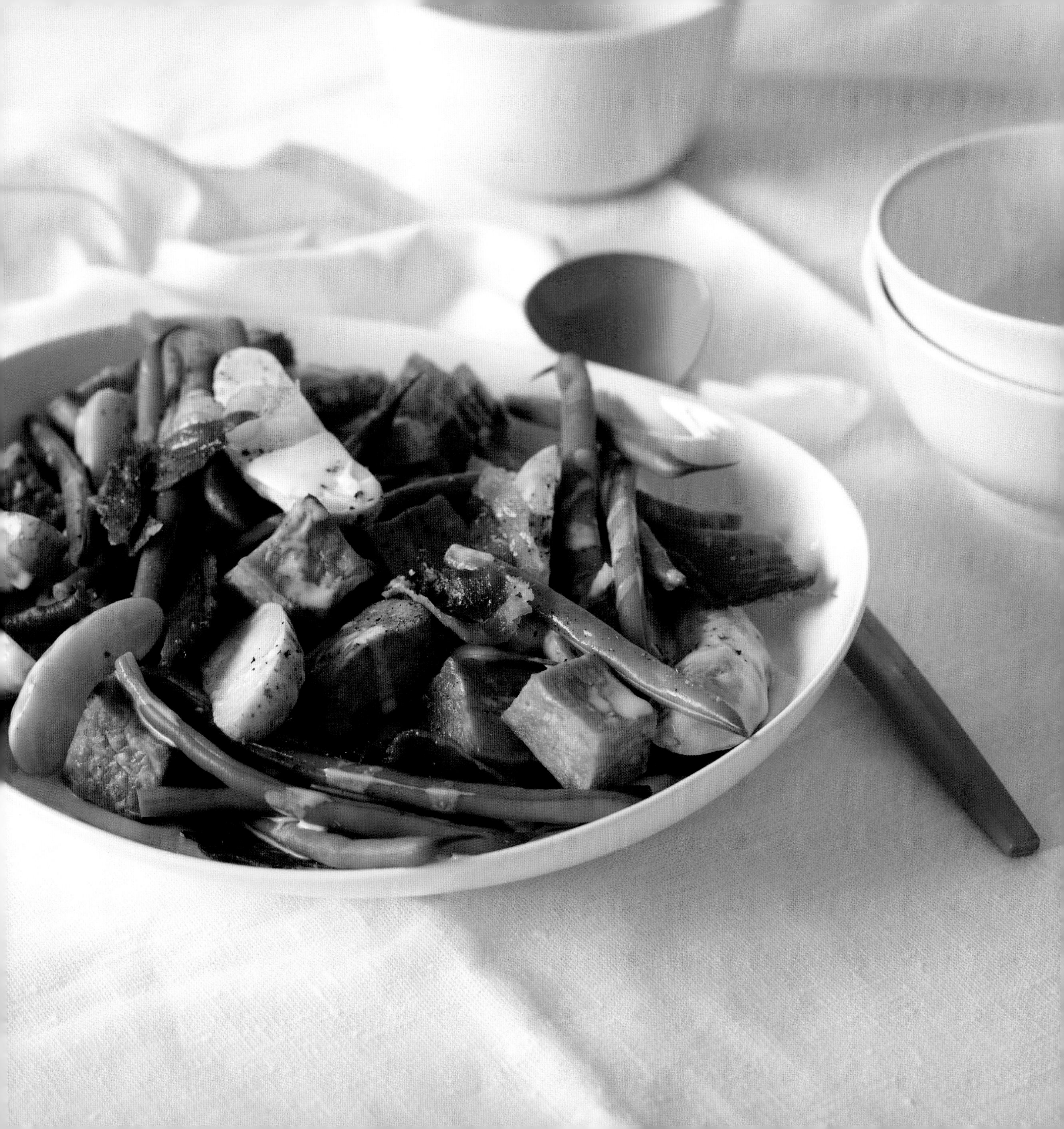

Fig and prosciutto salad with spiced quail

Five-spice powder is an aromatic spice blend that adds flavour without being too hot or peppery. I've used it here as part of a simple marinade for quail, adding an exotic note to this stylish dish.

SERVES 4

2 cloves garlic, crushed
1 teaspoon Chinese five-spice powder
1 tablespoon olive oil
salt and freshly ground black pepper
4 quails, breast and legs removed
2 teaspoons grated lemon zest
2 tablespoons extra virgin olive oil, plus extra for drizzling
100 g prosciutto, sliced
6 figs
3 cups (100 g) baby rocket leaves

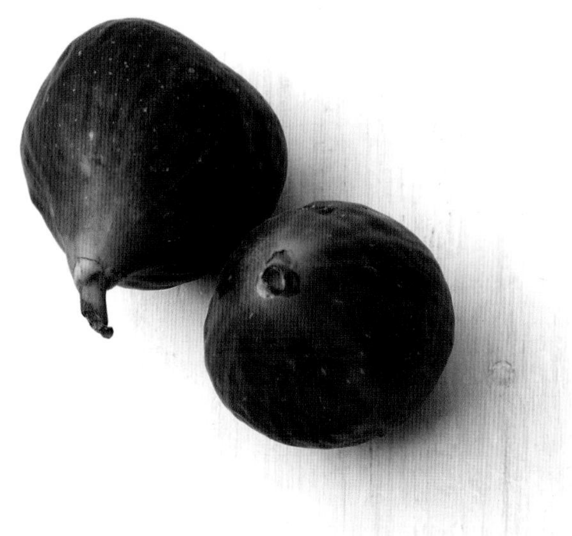

Combine the garlic, five-spice powder, olive oil, salt and pepper in a bowl and brush over the quail pieces. Place the quail in a baking dish, then cover and marinate in the fridge for 2–3 hours.

Place the lemon zest and extra virgin olive oil in a small screw-top jar and shake well to combine. Set aside to let the flavours infuse.

Preheat the oven to 180°C.

Place the prosciutto on a baking tray and bake for 10 minutes or until crisp. Set aside to cool, then break into pieces.

Cut the figs in half and place on another baking tray. Bake for 7–8 minutes or until slightly softened and warmed through. Remove and set aside.

Remove the quail pieces from the fridge and cover with foil. Bake for 20 minutes or until cooked through.

Combine the rocket, prosciutto and lemon-infused oil in a large bowl. Divide the rocket, prosciutto, fig halves and quail pieces among four plates and season to taste. Finish with a drizzle of olive oil and serve.

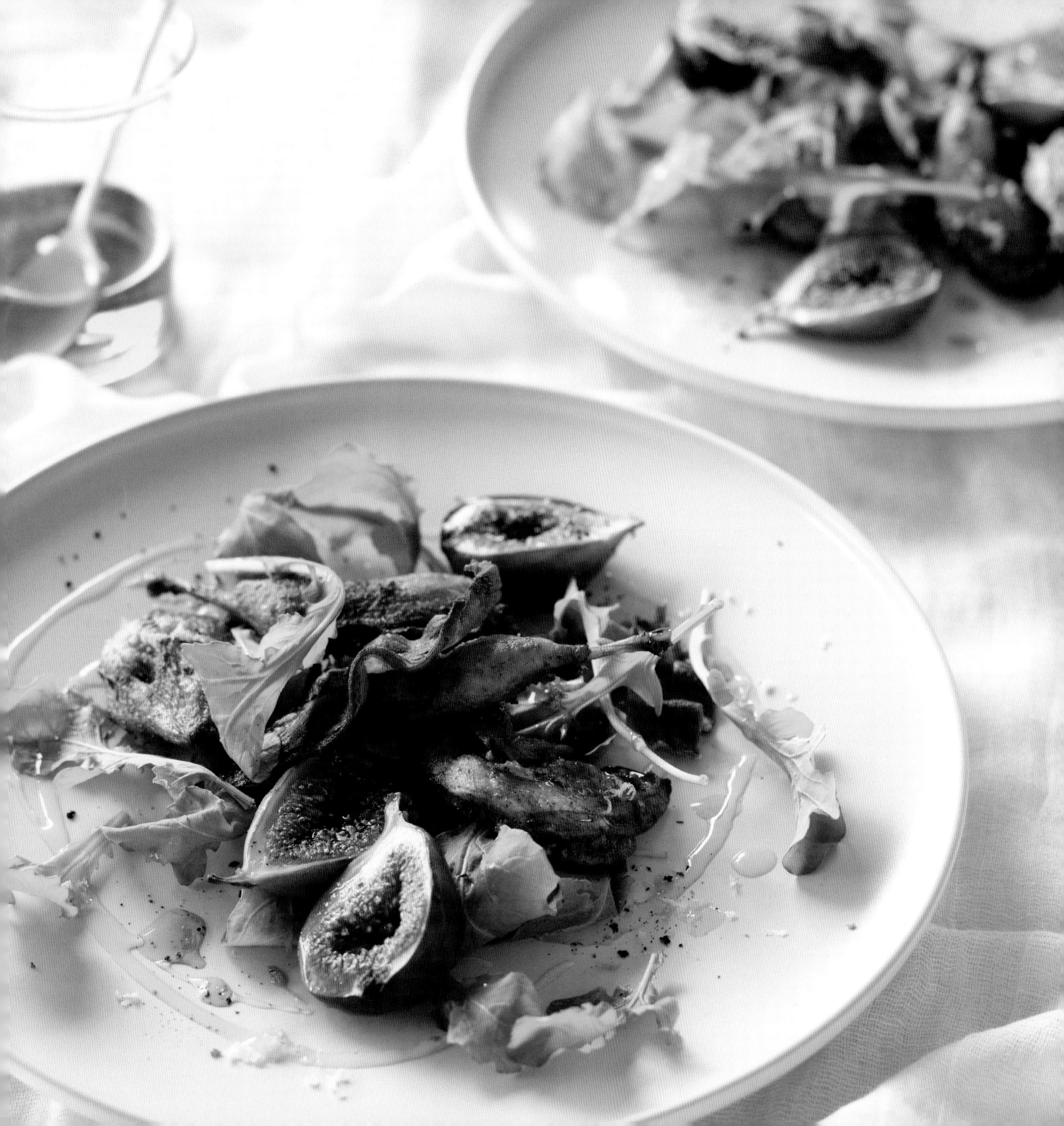

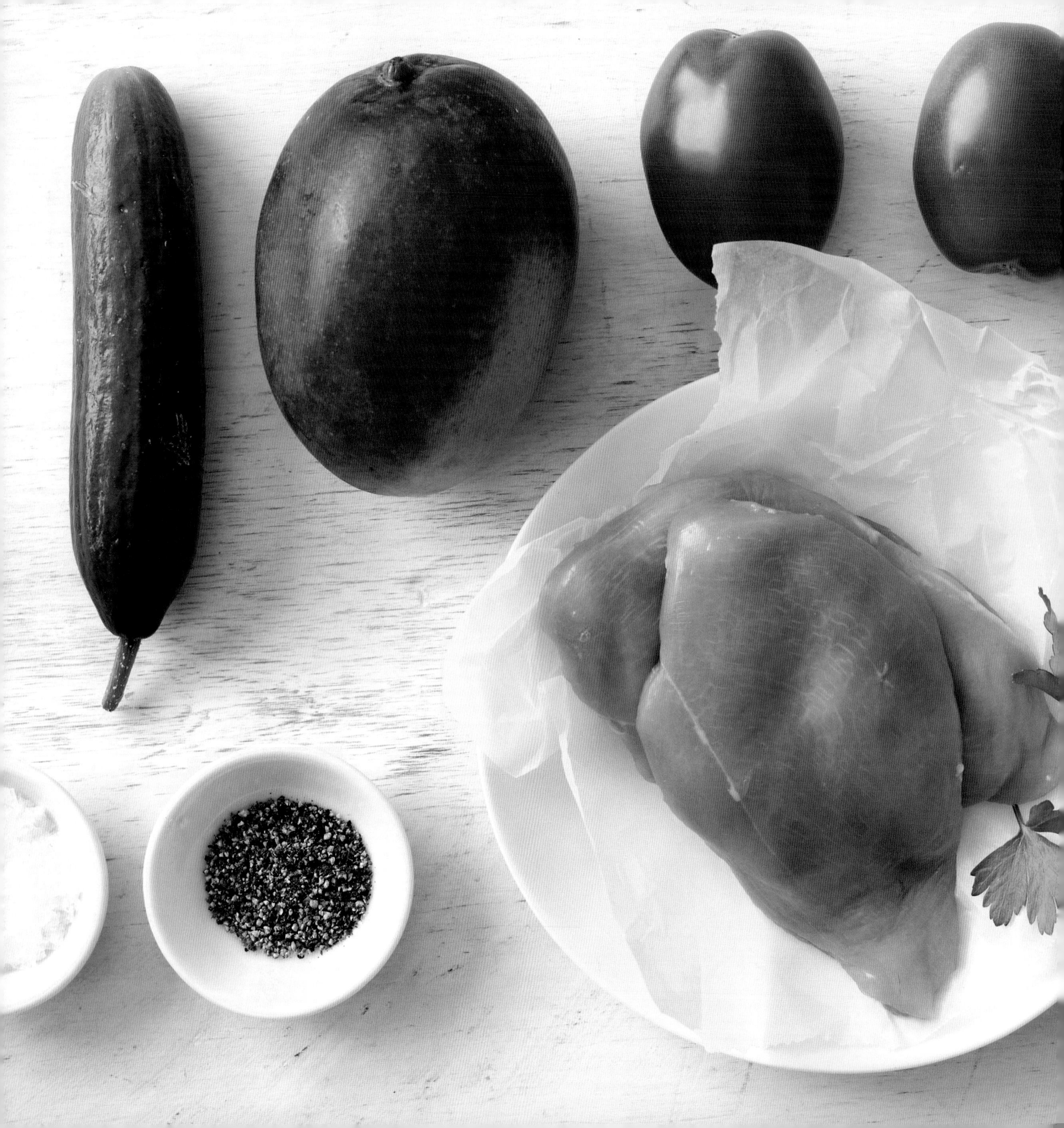

main meals with chicken

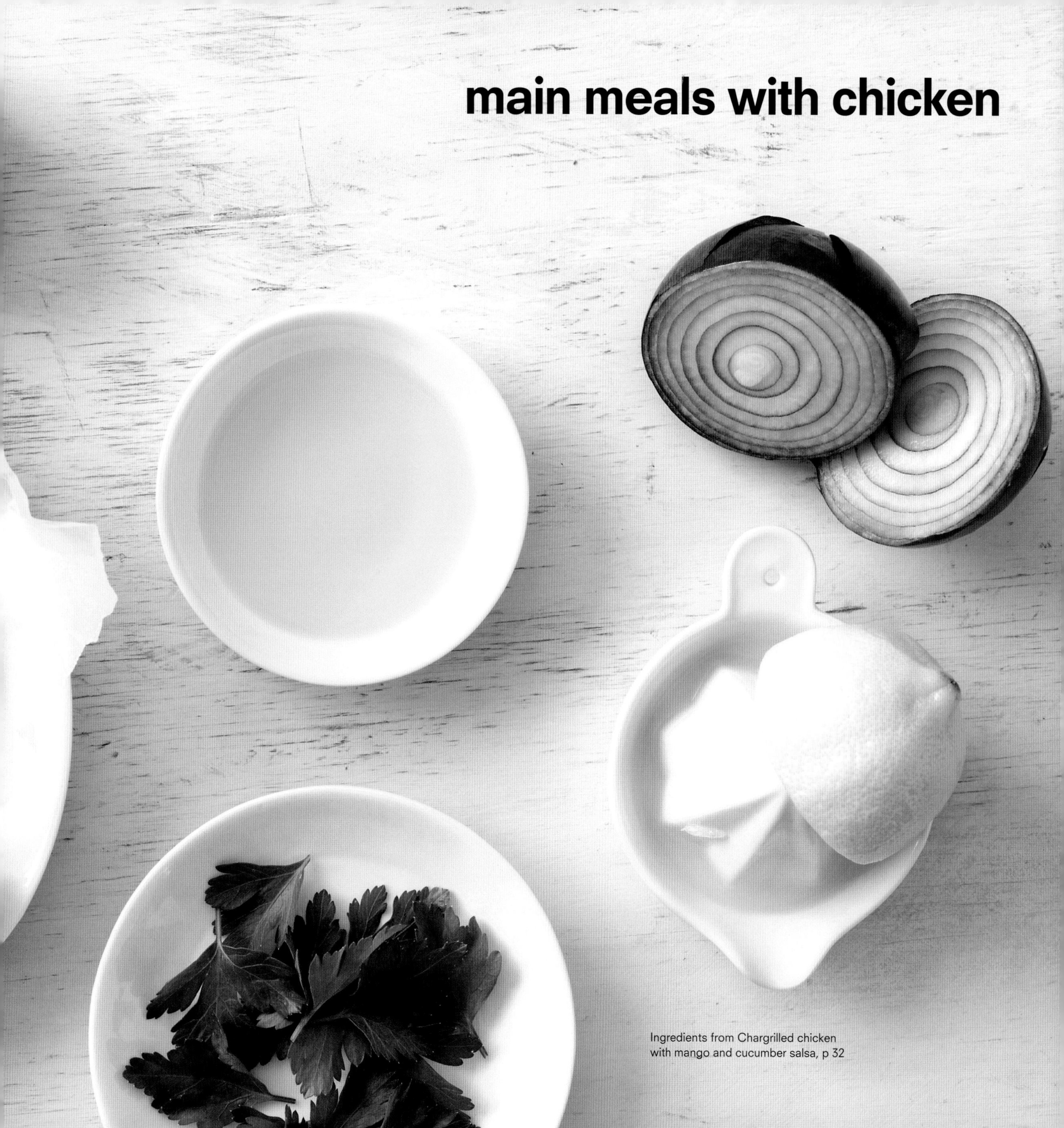

Ingredients from Chargrilled chicken with mango and cucumber salsa, p 32

Chargrilled chicken with mango and cucumber salsa

This is a great recipe for the warmer months, and may be cooked on the stovetop or barbecue. Chicken is delicious with the salsa, but you could also try it with chargrilled fish fillets, such as snapper. Enjoy it with pear and rocket salad (see page 22). SERVES 4

4 × 150 g skinless chicken breast fillets
1 tablespoon lemon juice
1 tablespoon olive oil
salt and freshly ground black pepper
baby rocket leaves, to serve

MANGO AND CUCUMBER SALSA
1 mango, diced
1 small cucumber, diced
1 small roma (plum) tomato, diced
¼ red onion, diced
1 tablespoon olive oil
2 teaspoons lemon juice
2 tablespoons finely chopped flat-leaf parsley
salt and freshly ground black pepper

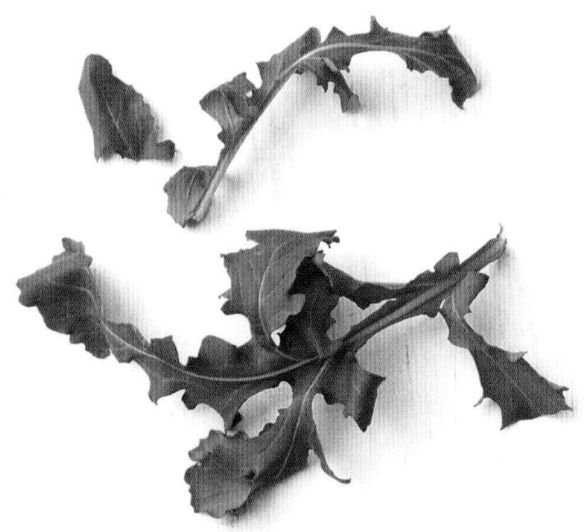

Place the chicken fillets in a non-metallic bowl, add the lemon juice, olive oil, salt and pepper and turn to coat. Cover and refrigerate for 2 hours.

To make the salsa, place the diced mango, cucumber, tomato and onion in a small bowl. Add the olive oil, lemon juice and parsley and stir to combine well. Season to taste with salt and pepper.

Heat a chargrill pan over medium–high heat. Add the chicken fillets and cook for 3–5 minutes each side, turning once only. Remove and allow to rest for a few minutes, then cut into slices.

Divide the chicken among four plates and scatter the salsa and rocket over the top.

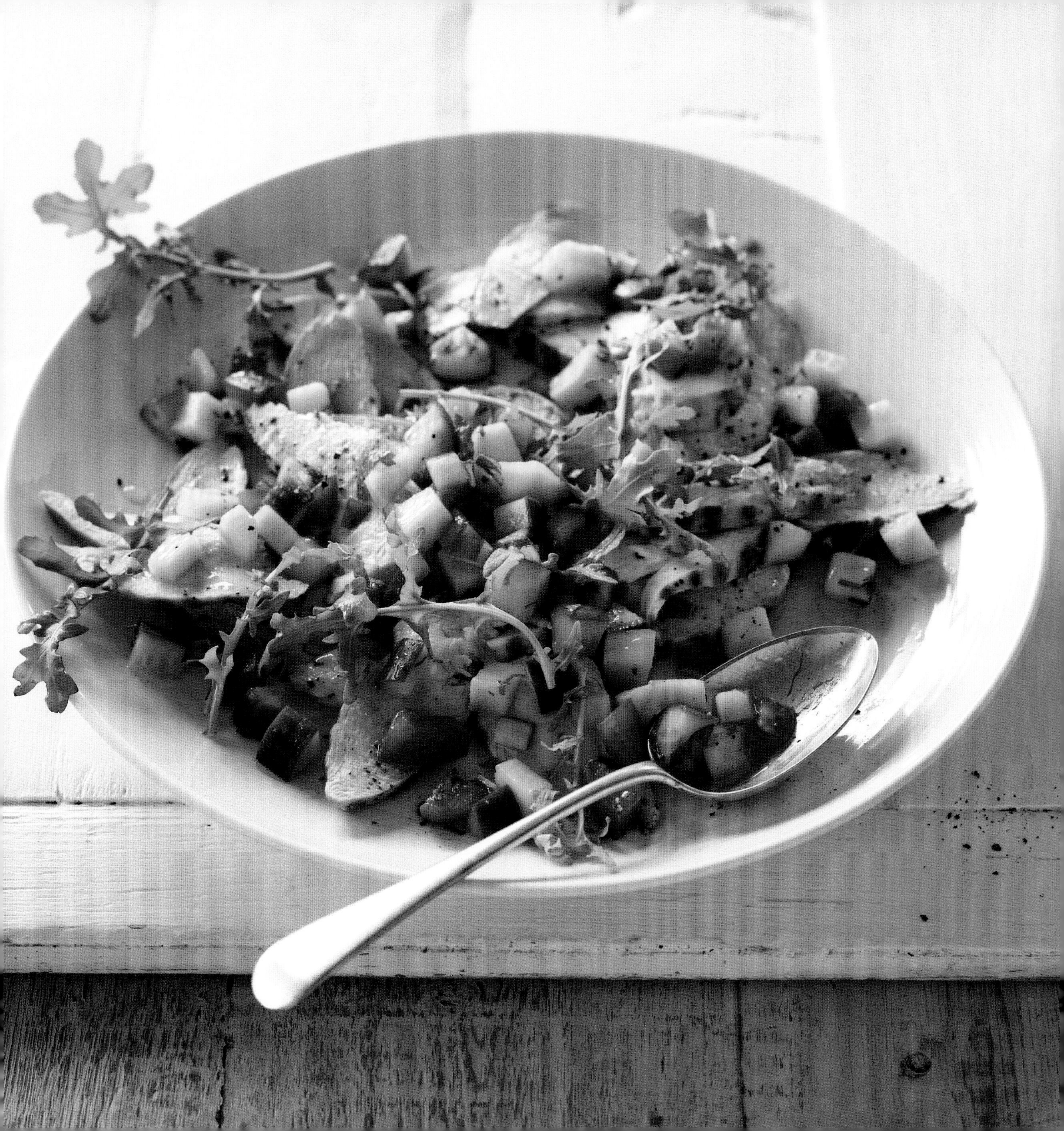

Chicken pilaf

Rice-based dishes are found in various incarnations in many cuisines: think risotto, paella, pilaf and fried rice. Here, the rice is simmered in spiced stock with chicken and vegetables to give a satisfying meal that will appeal to everyone. SERVES 4

1 teaspoon olive oil
1 clove garlic, crushed
1 onion, chopped
450 g skinless chicken breast fillet, diced
½–1 teaspoon chilli powder
1 teaspoon ground turmeric
3 cups (750 ml) gluten-free, wheat-free, dairy-free, soy-free chicken stock, plus extra if needed
400 g tin chopped tomatoes
1½ cups (300 g) long-grain rice
½ green capsicum (pepper), diced
½ red capsicum (pepper), diced
3 sticks celery, sliced
¾ cup (90 g) frozen peas
lemon wedges, to serve

Heat the olive oil in a large non-stick frying pan over medium–high heat. Add the garlic, onion, chicken, chilli and turmeric and cook until the chicken is nicely browned. Reduce the heat to medium–low, add the stock, chopped tomatoes and rice and simmer, covered, for 10 minutes.

Add the capsicum, celery and peas and simmer, stirring occasionally, for 15 minutes or until the rice is tender. Add a little more stock or water if necessary.

Spoon into shallow bowls and serve immediately with lemon wedges.

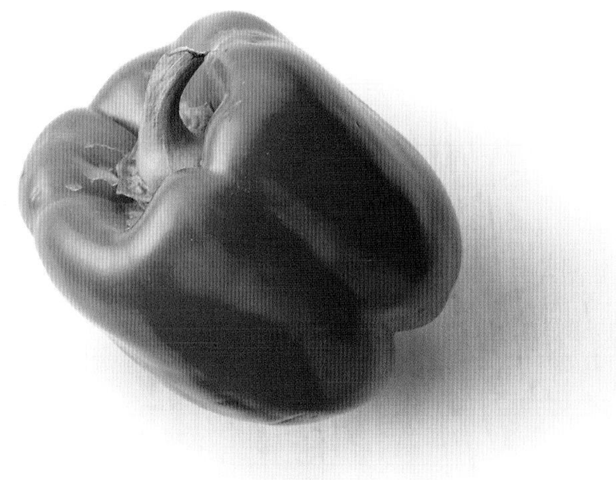

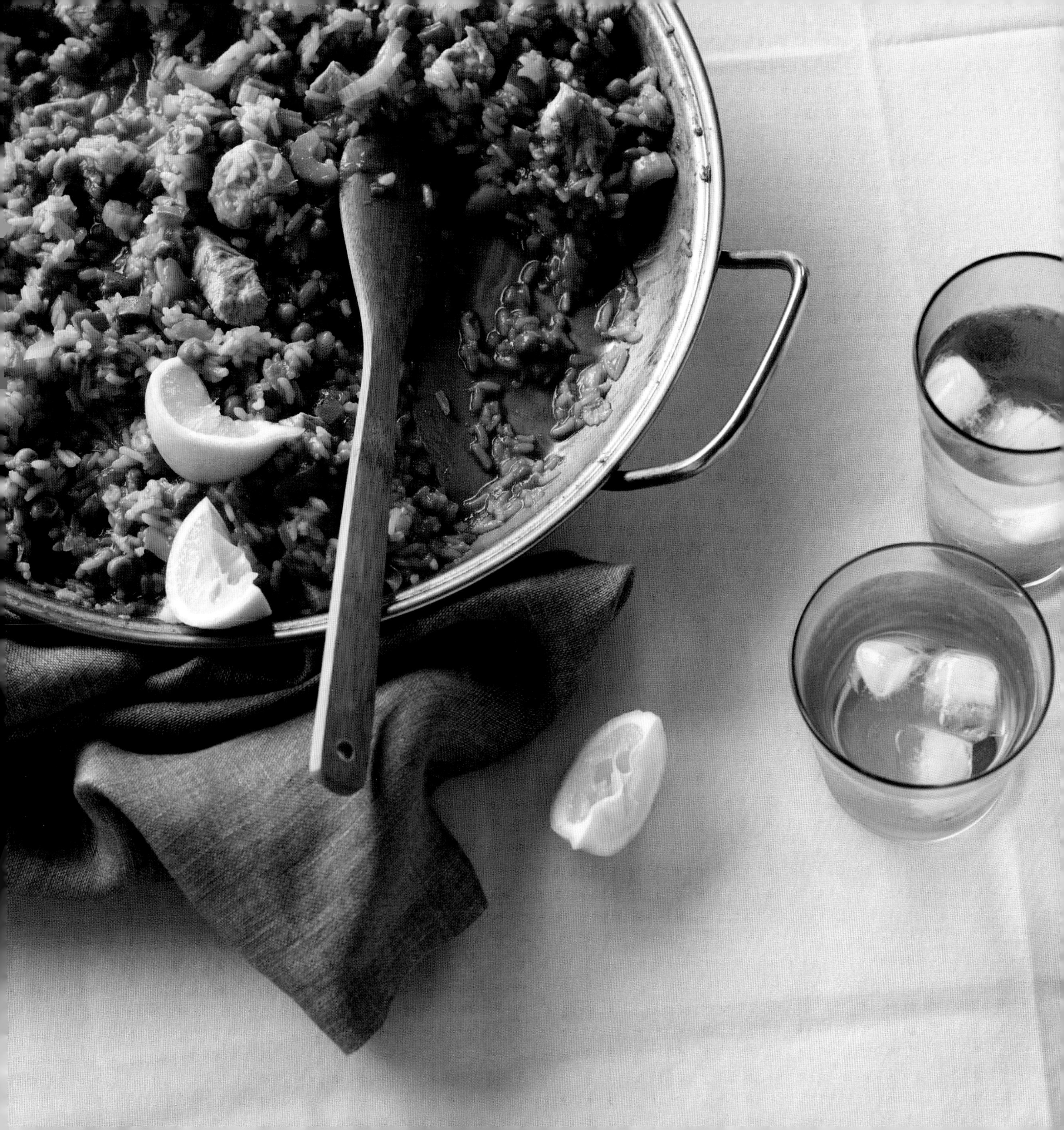

Smoked chicken pasta

I love to cook with smoked chicken as it adds a lovely depth of flavour. You can buy it in gourmet delicatessens and larger supermarkets. SERVES 4

350 g gluten-free, soy-free pasta*
3 tablespoons olive oil, plus extra to serve (optional)
2 cloves garlic, crushed
1 large smoked chicken fillet, sliced
50 g sundried tomatoes, drained and roughly chopped
2 cups (60 g) baby spinach leaves
salt and freshly ground black pepper

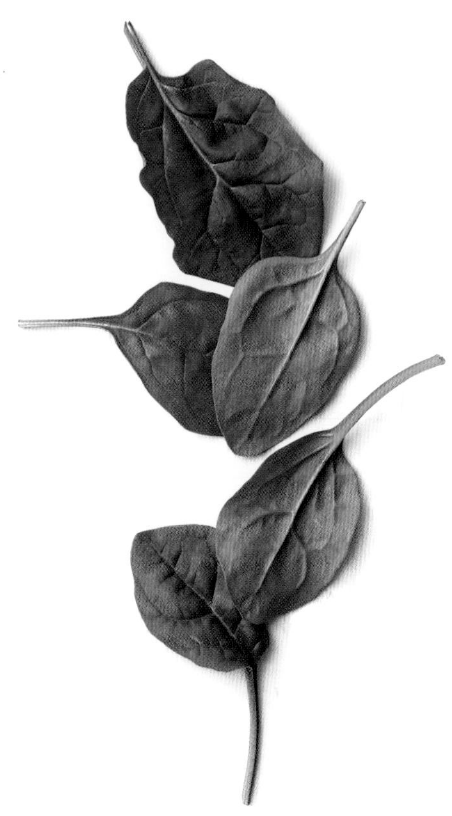

Cook the pasta in a large saucepan of boiling water until just tender. Drain and return to the pan, then stir through 2 tablespoons olive oil. Cover and keep warm.

Meanwhile, heat the remaining olive oil in a large frying pan over medium heat. Add the garlic, chicken and sundried tomatoes and cook until the chicken is golden. Add the pasta and toss over medium heat until warmed through. Stir through the spinach leaves, then season to taste with salt and pepper and serve with an extra drizzle of olive oil, if desired.

***For egg allergy**
Use egg-free pasta.

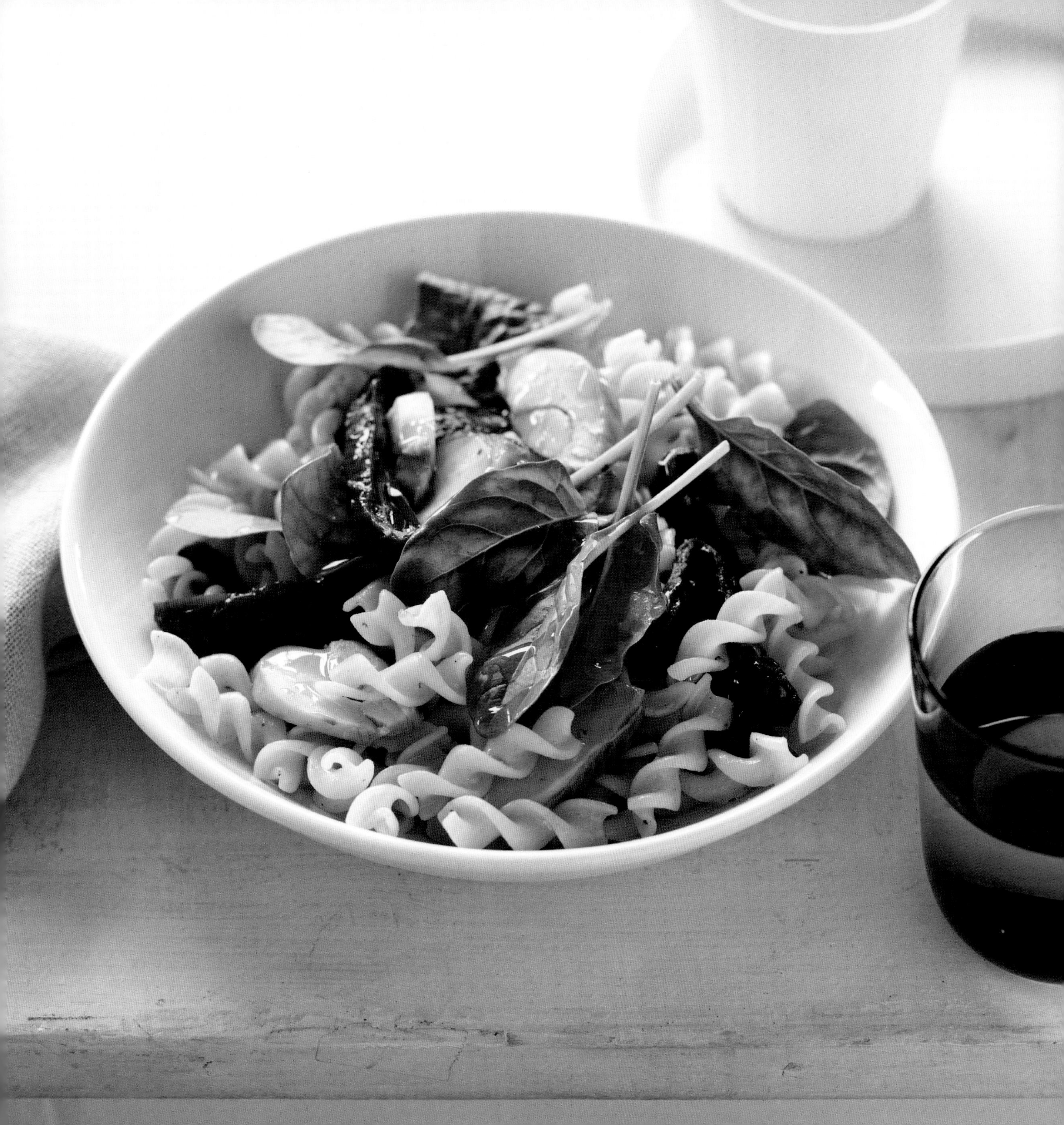

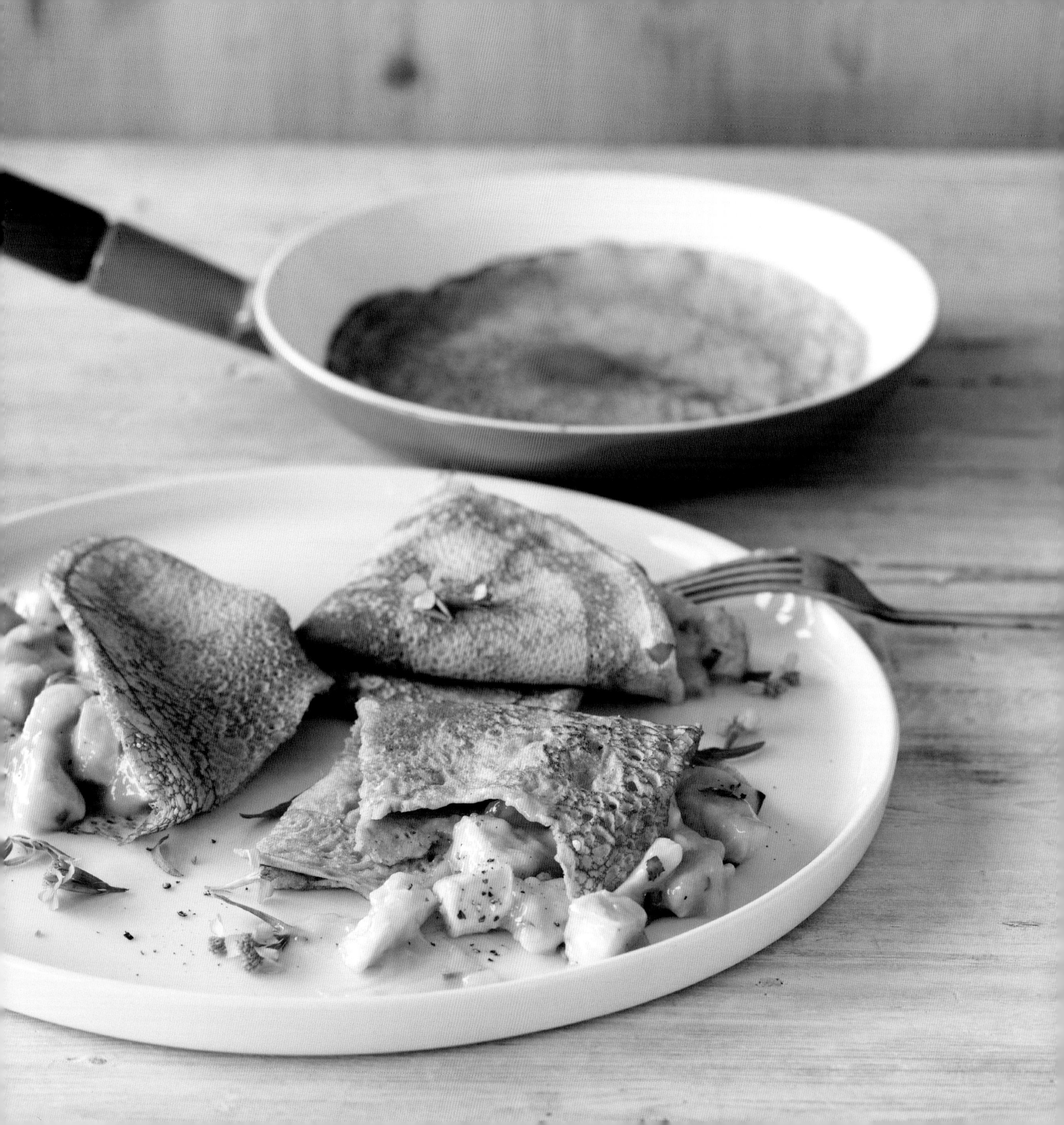

Buckwheat crepes with chicken and tarragon filling

Contrary to what you might think, buckwheat has no wheat in it at all and, when ground to a flour, makes a delicious, nutty addition to crepes. Tarragon is used in many French dishes, and goes beautifully with the chicken in this filling.

SERVES 4

¾ cup (100 g) fine rice flour
⅔ cup (135 g) buckwheat flour
¾ teaspoon bicarbonate of soda
1½ cups (375 ml) rice milk
1 egg, lightly beaten*
1 tablespoon soy-free, dairy-free spread, melted
cooking spray
green salad and edible flowers, to serve (optional)

CHICKEN AND TARRAGON FILLING
olive oil, for pan-frying
450 g skinless chicken breast fillet, finely diced
2½ tablespoons maize cornflour
2 cups (500 ml) rice milk
1 tablespoon chopped tarragon
salt and freshly ground black pepper

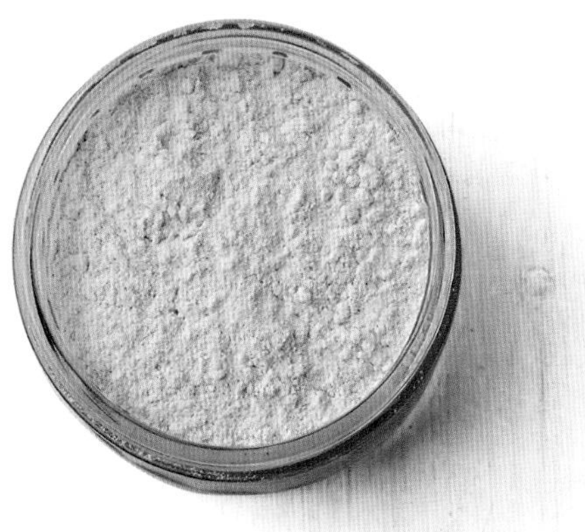

Sift the flours and bicarbonate of soda into a bowl. Add the rice milk and egg and blend to form a smooth batter. Stir in the melted dairy-free spread, then cover with plastic film and set aside for 20 minutes.

Heat a 22 cm non-stick frying pan over medium heat and spray with cooking spray. Pour in 3–4 tablespoons batter and tilt to coat the base of the pan. Cook until bubbles appear on the surface, then turn and cook the other side for a minute or so. Remove to a plate and keep warm. Repeat with the remaining batter to make eight crepes altogether.

To make the filling, heat a little olive oil in a small, deep frying pan over medium heat and cook the chicken pieces until golden brown. Remove from the pan. In a small bowl, combine the cornflour with 3 tablespoons rice milk to make a paste. Add the remaining rice milk, mixing well until smooth, then pour into the pan with the chicken juices and stir over medium heat until thickened. Don't let the mixture boil. Add the tarragon and chicken, season to taste and stir until well combined.

Divide the filling among the crepes. Fold or roll up and serve with edible flowers and salad, if liked.

***For egg allergy**
Place 2 teaspoons psyllium husks in a small bowl and pour over ½ cup (125 ml) boiling water, stirring constantly to ensure the psyllium does not clump together. Set aside for 4–5 minutes until it forms a gel, stirring occasionally. Use in place of the egg.

Chicken and corn soup

This comforting soup is made with leg and thigh portions of chicken, but you could also use other cuts. A chicken carcass is fine to make the broth, but you'll need to add three or four thigh fillets to make sure there is enough meat in the soup. SERVES 4

2 teaspoons canola oil
1 onion, diced
4 skinless chicken leg and thigh portions
2 litres gluten-free, wheat-free, dairy-free, soy-free chicken stock
2 × 420 g tins gluten-free, wheat-free creamed corn
¾ cup (150 g) white rice
salt and freshly ground black pepper
coriander leaves, to garnish (optional)

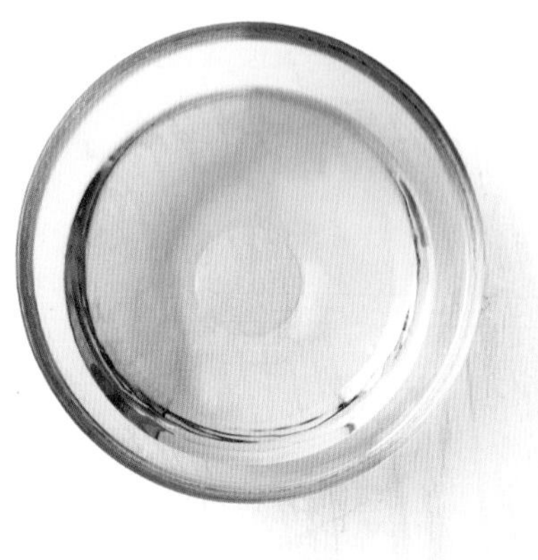

Heat the canola oil in a large stockpot over medium–high heat, add the onion and cook until softened. Add the chicken pieces and pour in the stock. Cover and bring to the boil, then reduce the heat to medium–low and simmer for 20 minutes.

Remove the chicken pieces from the pot and set aside to cool slightly. Remove the meat from the bones and finely shred it.

Return the chicken to the pot and stir in the corn and rice. Simmer over medium–low heat for 20 minutes or until the rice is tender. Season to taste and serve garnished with coriander leaves, if liked.

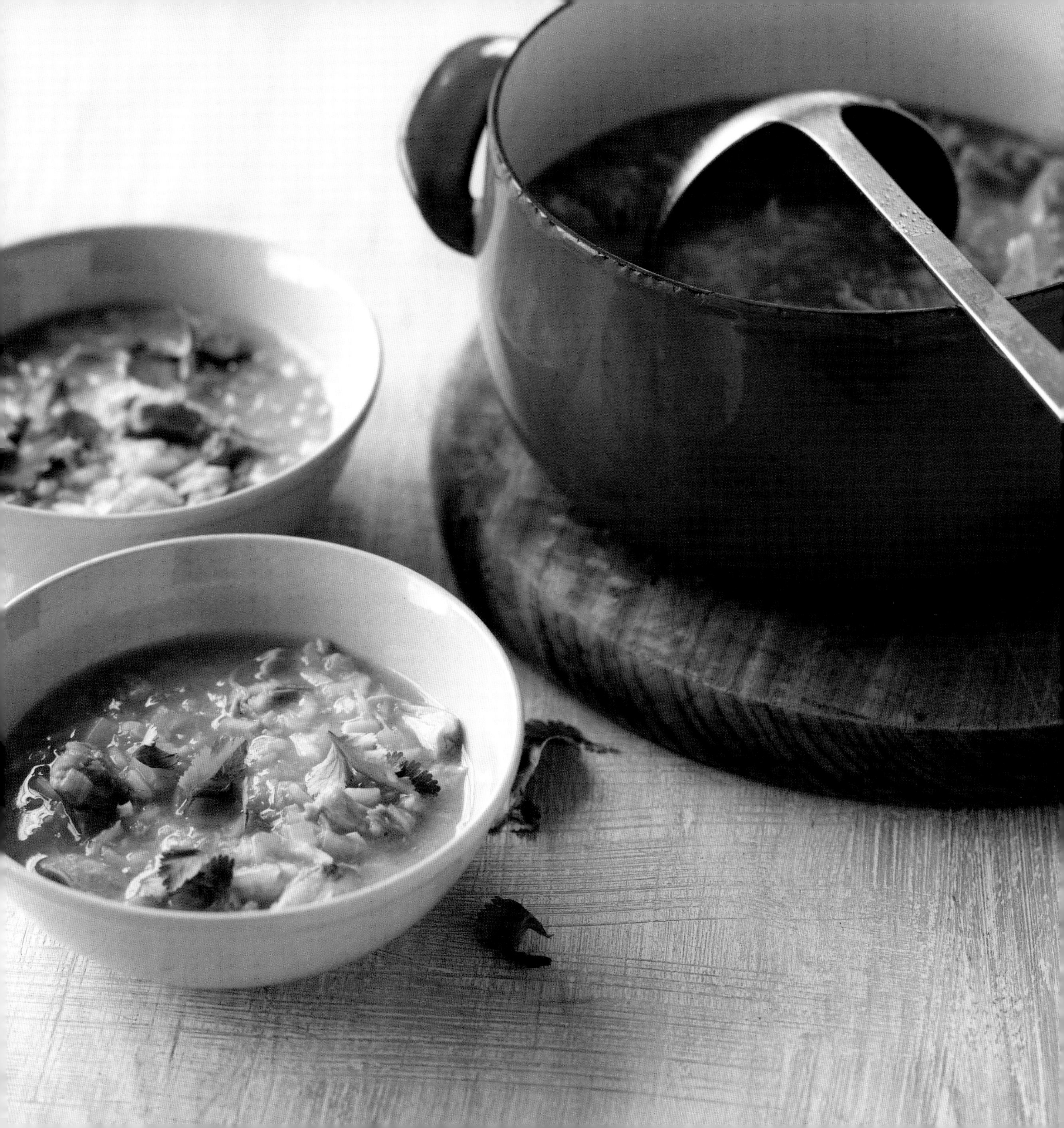

Chicken with chilli caramel sauce

The recipe name alone tends to get people's attention, and I'm happy to say the dish delivers on flavour too. The unusual combination of spicy chilli and sweet caramel is just perfect with chicken.

SERVES 4

4 × 150 g skinless chicken breast fillets
1 tablespoon olive oil
80 g soy-free, dairy-free spread
2 cloves garlic, crushed
2 tablespoons brown sugar
½–1 teaspoon finely chopped red chilli
salad or vegetables, to serve

MARINADE
1 clove garlic, crushed
1 tablespoon olive oil
1 tablespoon lemon juice
freshly ground black pepper

Place the chicken fillets in a non-metallic bowl, add the marinade ingredients and turn to coat. Cover and refrigerate for 3–4 hours.

Heat the olive oil in a large frying pan over medium–low heat. Add the chicken and cook for 3–5 minutes each side or until just cooked and golden brown. Remove from the pan, then cover and leave to rest while you make the sauce.

Melt the dairy-free spread in a small frying pan over medium–low heat. Add the garlic, brown sugar and chilli and cook for 2–3 minutes or until the sugar has melted and the sauce is beginning to caramelise.

Place a chicken breast on each plate, pour the sauce over the top and serve with your choice of salad or vegetables.

Chicken with sage 'butter' sauce >

Sage is the hero here so make sure you use fresh leaves rather than dried sage. If you can't find any, fresh thyme, marjoram, rosemary or chives would also work well.

SERVES 4

4 × 150 g skinless chicken breast fillets
80 g soy-free, dairy-free spread
2 cloves garlic, extra, thinly sliced
20 sage leaves
salad or vegetables, to serve

MARINADE
1 clove garlic, crushed
1 tablespoon lemon juice
1 tablespoon olive oil
salt and freshly ground black pepper

Place the chicken fillets in a non-metallic bowl, add the marinade ingredients and turn to coat. Cover and refrigerate for 2 hours.

Melt 1 tablespoon dairy-free spread in a large frying pan over medium heat, add the chicken fillets and cook for 3–5 minutes each side or until just cooked and golden brown. Thickly slice each fillet, then place on warmed serving dishes and cover with foil.

In the same pan, melt the remaining dairy-free spread over medium–low heat until foaming. Add the extra garlic and sage leaves and cook until crisp but not burnt, stirring regularly. Take off the heat immediately and pour over the chicken. Season to taste and serve with your choice of salad or vegetables.

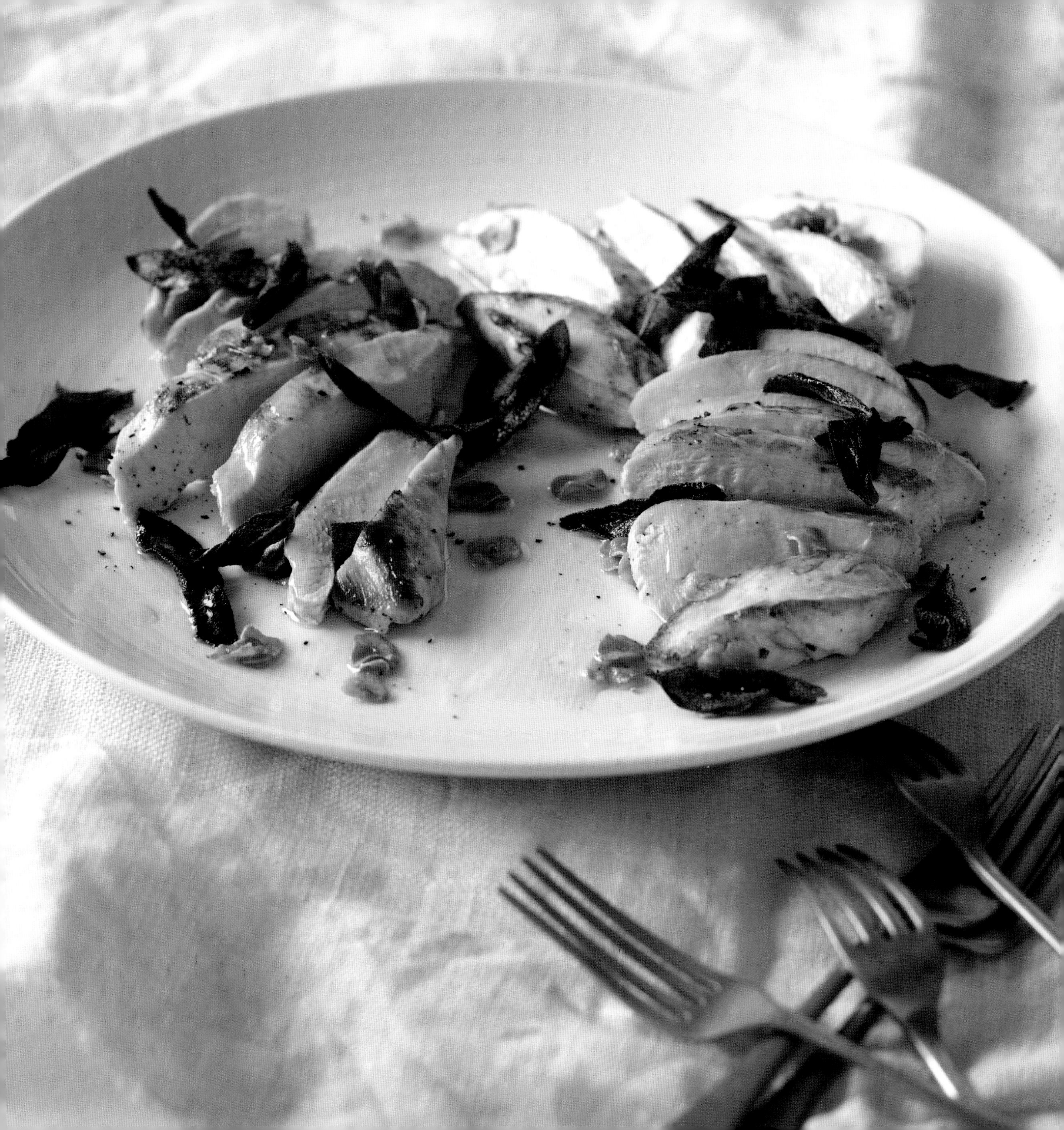

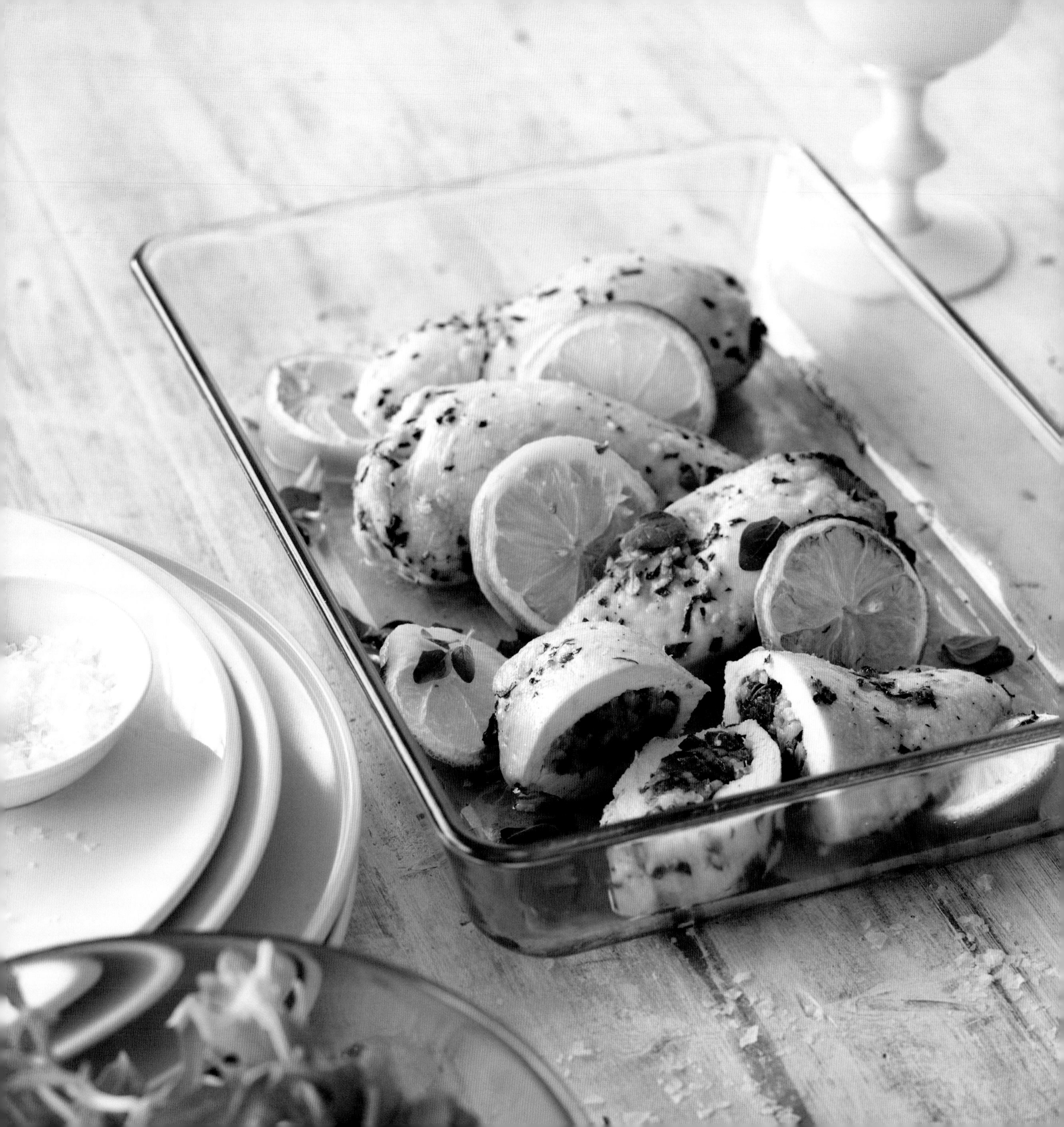

Mediterranean chicken pockets

This recipe is a great way to use up leftover cooked rice. If you don't have any to hand, you'll need to cook about ⅓ cup (65 g) uncooked rice to make the right quantity.

SERVES 4

4 × 150 g skinless chicken breast fillets
3 tablespoons olive oil
1 clove garlic, crushed
1 teaspoon chopped oregano, plus extra leaves to garnish
1 teaspoon finely grated lemon zest
1 lemon, thickly sliced
salad, to serve

FILLING

⅔ cup (100 g) sundried tomatoes in oil, drained and finely chopped
1 cup (70 g) cooked white rice
1 tablespoon finely grated lemon zest
1 tablespoon chopped oregano
salt and freshly ground black pepper

Preheat the oven to 180°C.

Using a small sharp knife, cut into the thickest part of each chicken fillet to form an internal pocket (you want to cut from the middle to about 1 cm from the edge).

To make the filling, combine all the ingredients in a bowl. Spoon into the chicken pockets, pressing it in firmly and making sure it is evenly spread. Seal the ends with a toothpick.

Mix together the olive oil, garlic, oregano and lemon zest in a small bowl and brush over the chicken pieces. Place in a baking tray, add the lemon slices and bake for 20 minutes or until golden brown. Remove from the oven and rest, covered, for 5–10 minutes. Cut into 2 cm thick slices and serve with salad. The chicken may also be served cold on a platter.

Quick Thai chicken risotto

Traditionally, risotto is made by gradually adding hot stock to the rice and stirring between additions until all the liquid has been absorbed. This recipe adds all the stock at once, yet still achieves the perfect risotto texture. Try it for yourself. If you are allergic to coconut, replace the coconut milk with rice milk. SERVES 4

1 tablespoon olive oil
1 onion, finely chopped
2 cloves garlic, crushed
2 × 250 g skinless chicken breast fillets, sliced
1.25 litres gluten-free, wheat-free, dairy-free, soy-free chicken stock
1⅓ cups (265 g) arborio rice
1–2 tablespoons gluten-free, wheat-free, dairy-free, soy-free, crustacean-free Thai yellow curry paste
⅓ cup (80 ml) coconut milk
2 cups (60 g) baby spinach leaves
140 g tin sliced bamboo shoots, drained
salt and freshly ground black pepper
2 tablespoons finely chopped coriander

Heat the olive oil in a medium frying pan over medium heat, add the onion and garlic and cook until softened. Add the chicken pieces and cook until golden brown and cooked through. Remove the pan from the heat.

Pour the stock into a large heavy-based saucepan and bring to the boil over medium–high heat. Reduce the heat to medium–low and add the rice and curry paste. Cook, stirring regularly, for about 15 minutes or until all the liquid has been absorbed and the rice is tender. Stir in the chicken mixture, coconut milk, spinach and bamboo shoots. Season to taste with salt and pepper, then spoon into four bowls, sprinkle with coriander and serve.

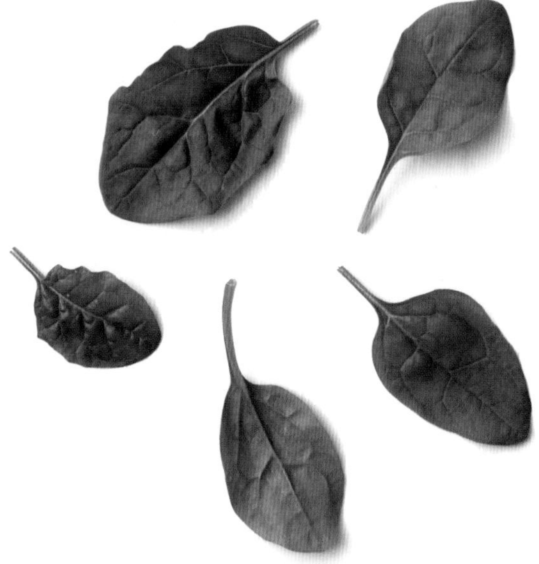

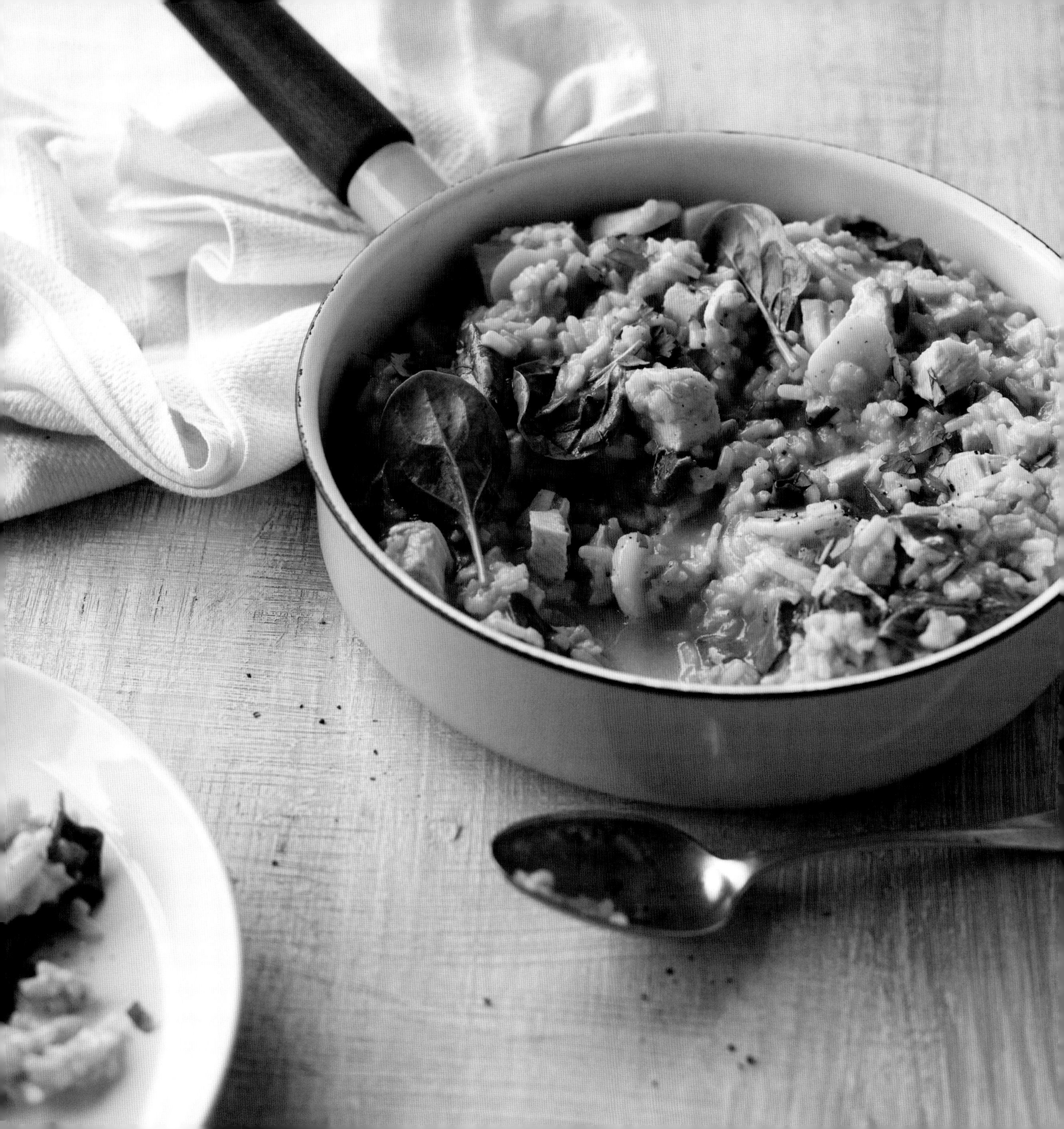

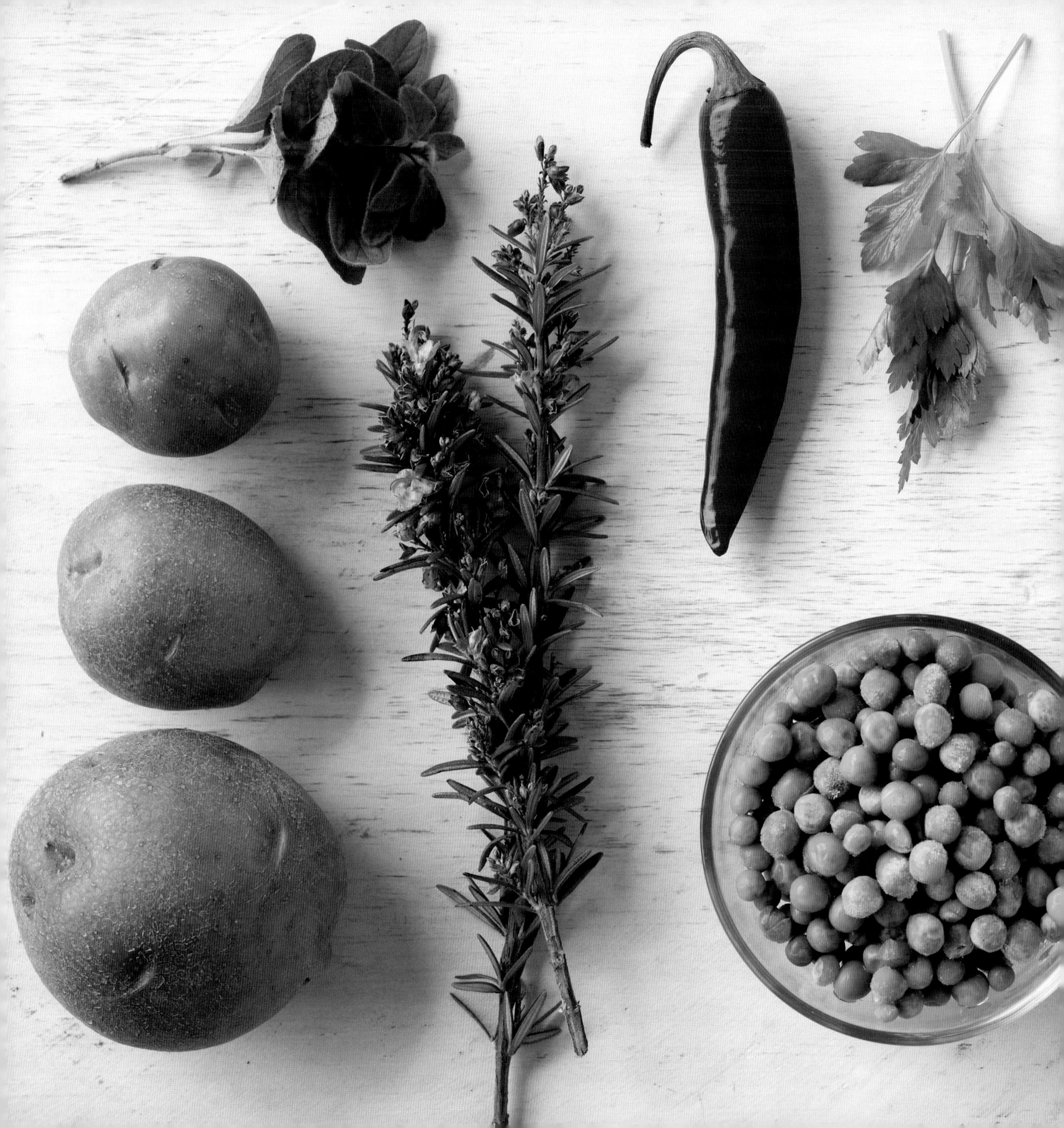

main meals with meat

Ingredients from Herb-crusted rack of lamb with minted pea puree, p 51

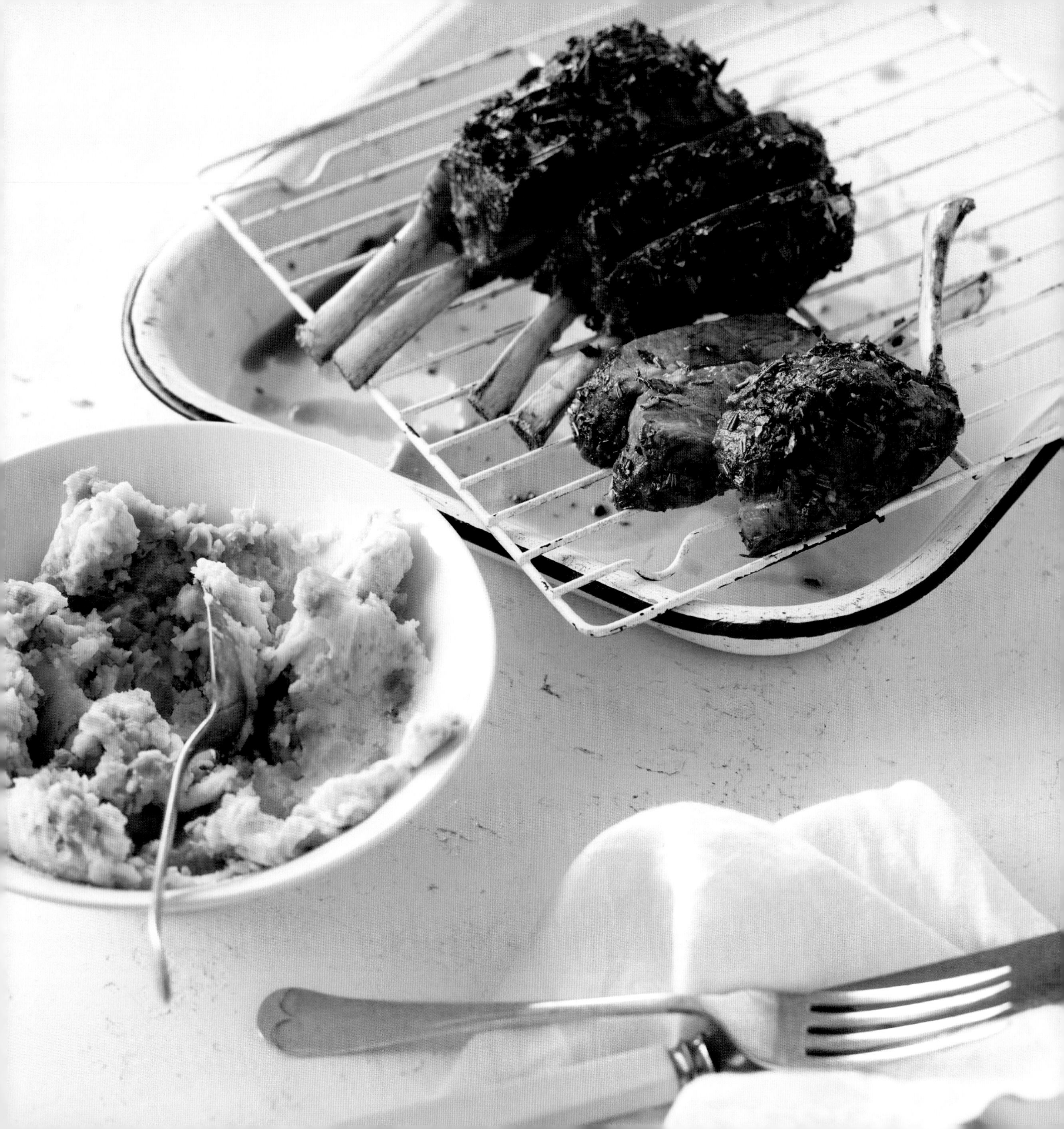

Herb-crusted rack of lamb with minted pea puree

It's hard to beat fresh herbs with roast lamb, and as mint is a natural partner for both lamb and peas, the minted pea puree is the perfect side dish. SERVES 4

3 tablespoons oregano leaves
4 tablespoons flat-leaf parsley leaves
1 tablespoon rosemary leaves
1 large red chilli, chopped (optional)
3 cloves garlic, crushed
3 tablespoons olive oil
salt and freshly ground black pepper
4 racks of 4 lamb cutlets, trimmed of fat

MINTED PEA PUREE
1 large potato, diced
1 cup (120 g) frozen peas
2 tablespoons soy-free, dairy-free spread
3 tablespoons rice milk
2 tablespoons mint leaves
salt and freshly ground black pepper

Preheat the oven to 180°C.

Combine the herbs, chilli (if using), garlic, olive oil, salt and pepper in a small bowl. Rub the herb mixture over the lamb cutlets. Place in a baking dish and bake for 30 minutes or until the lamb is medium–rare.

Meanwhile, to make the minted pea puree, bring a small saucepan of water to the boil. Reduce the heat to medium, add the potato and cook, covered, until just tender. Add the peas and cook for a further 5 minutes. Drain, then mash with a potato masher with the dairy spread, rice milk and mint leaves. Season to taste with salt and pepper.

Cut each rack into two-cutlet pieces. Serve two pieces per person with the minted pea puree.

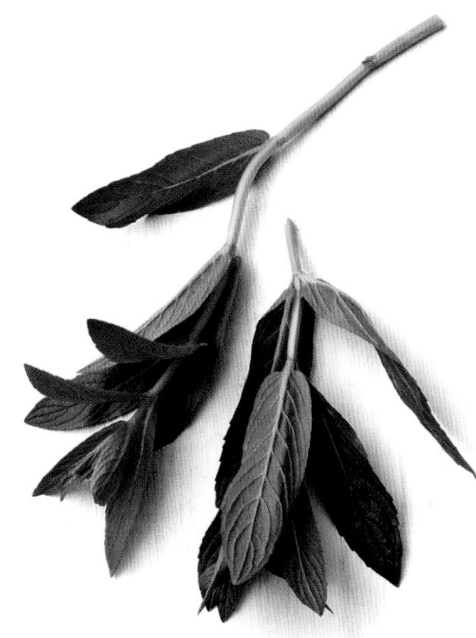

Beef with herb 'butter'

Rib-eye steaks (also called scotch fillet) are a tender cut of beef, making them easy to cook. Alternatively, you could use T-bone or porterhouse steaks. SERVES 4

1 tablespoon olive oil
1 tablespoon lemon juice
2 cloves garlic, crushed
salt and freshly ground black pepper
4 × 200 g rib-eye steaks
herbed wedges (see page 116), to serve (optional)
salad or vegetables, to serve

HERB 'BUTTER'
2 tablespoons chopped flat-leaf parsley
3 tablespoons finely chopped chives
100 g soy-free, dairy-free spread
salt and freshly ground black pepper

Combine the olive oil, lemon juice, garlic, salt and pepper in a non-metallic bowl. Add the steaks and turn to coat well, then cover and refrigerate for 2–3 hours.

To make the herb 'butter', place the herbs and dairy-free spread in a small bowl and mix together well. Season to taste, then return to the fridge to firm up. When firm, scoop out of the bowl onto a 15 cm × 15 cm sheet of foil and form into a log approximately 3 cm wide. Wrap in the foil and roll the log on the benchtop to refine the shape. Place in the freezer to firm up again.

Preheat a grill plate, chargrill pan or barbecue to medium–high and cook the steaks to your liking. Cover and leave to rest for a few minutes.

Remove the herb 'butter' from the freezer. Remove the foil and cut into 5 mm thick slices. Divide the steaks among warmed plates and top with a slice or two of herb 'butter'. Finish with a grinding of pepper, then serve with wedges, if liked, and your choice of salad or vegetables.

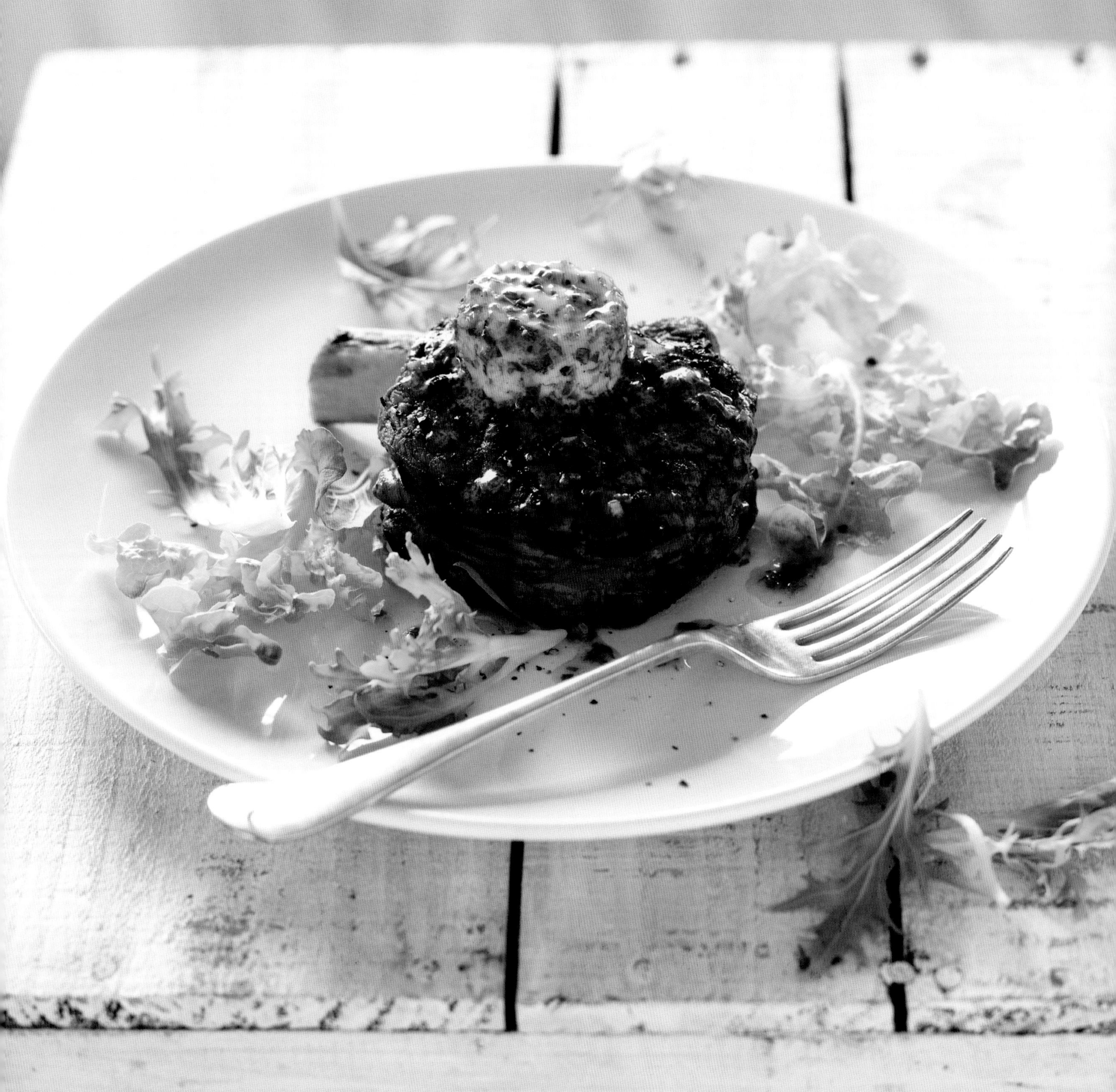

Lamb shank and vegetable soup

I love a thick vegetable soup, and not just during winter. This hearty soup is good on the day you make it, but tastes even better after a day or two when the flavours have had a chance to meld. Make sure you leave some for leftovers!

SERVES 6

1 tablespoon olive oil
3 medium lamb shanks
1 onion, chopped
1 clove garlic, crushed
1 kg pumpkin (squash), peeled, seeded and cut into 2 cm dice
3 carrots, halved, and cut into 1 cm dice
3 sticks celery, trimmed and cut into 1 cm thick slices
1.5 litres gluten-free, wheat-free, dairy-free, soy-free beef stock
salt and freshly ground black pepper
flat-leaf parsley leaves, to garnish

Heat the olive oil in a large stockpot over medium heat. Add the lamb shanks and cook until lightly browned on all sides. Remove and set aside on a plate. Add the onion and garlic to the pan and cook in the oil and meat juices for 2–3 minutes or until lightly browned. Add the pumpkin, carrot and celery and cook until lightly golden.

Pour in the stock and return the lamb shanks to the pan. Increase the heat to medium–high and bring to the boil, then reduce the heat and simmer, stirring occasionally, for 1 hour.

Take out the shanks and cool slightly, then remove the meat from the bones and cut into bite-sized chunks. Return the lamb to the soup and stir until well combined, breaking up the pumpkin pieces as you go. Season with salt and pepper, scatter over some parsley leaves and serve.

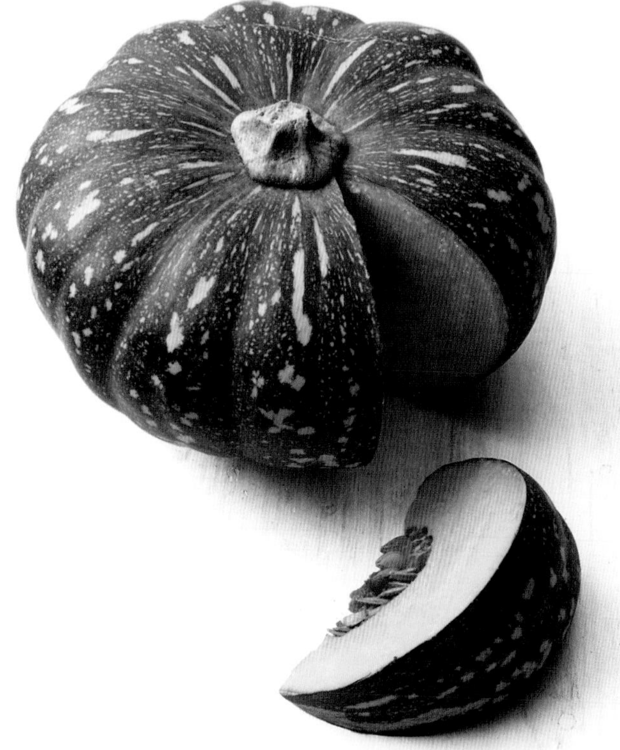

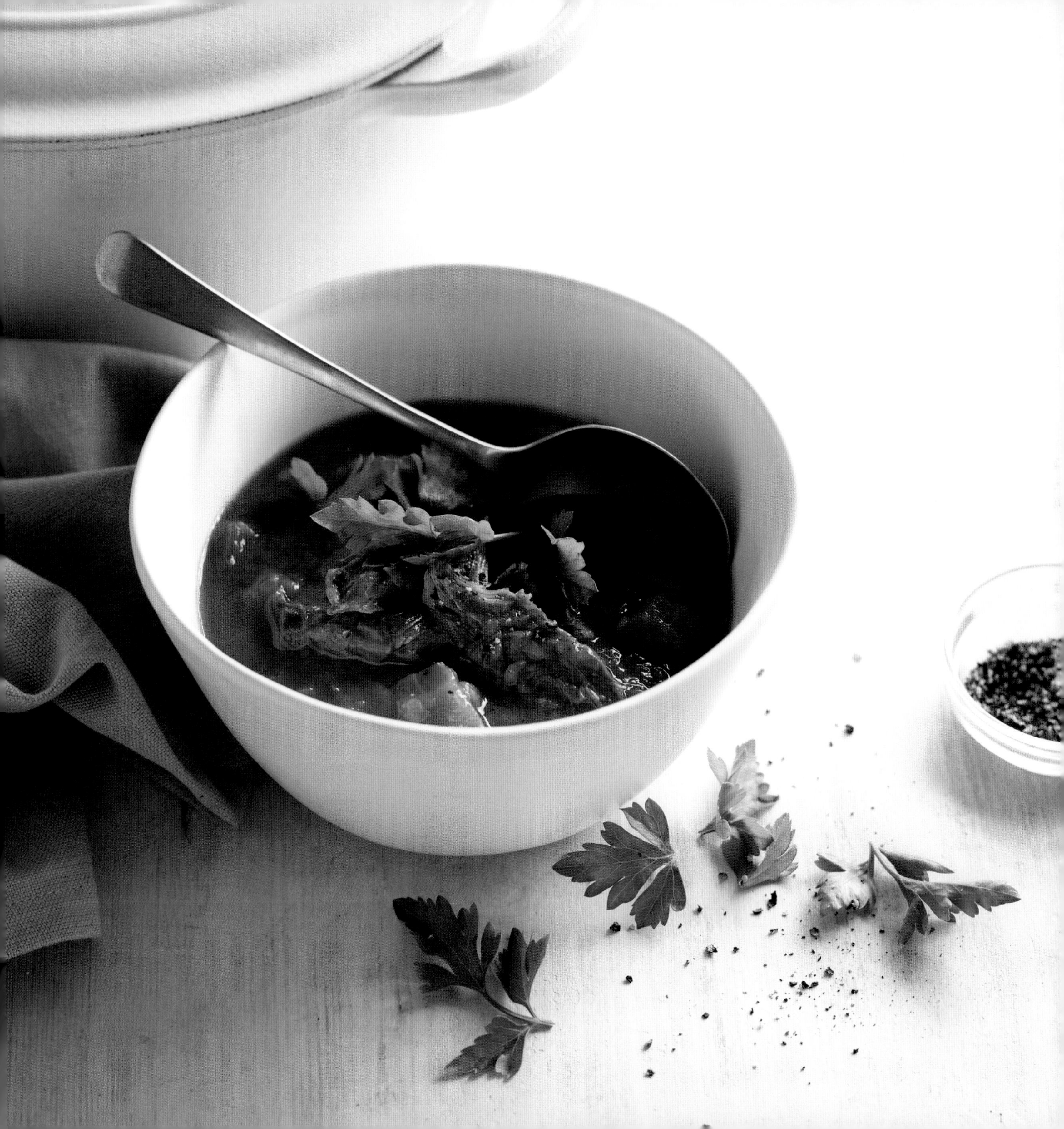

Chilli con carne

There are many variations on chilli con carne – this recipe is quick and simple to prepare and uses ingredients that are easy to find. A warming winter dish that's on the table in no time. SERVES 4

1 tablespoon canola oil
1 tablespoon ground cumin
1 teaspoon chilli powder (or to taste)
½ small onion, chopped
2 cloves garlic, crushed
600 g lean minced beef
1 × 400 g tin diced tomatoes
3 tablespoons tomato paste (puree)
1 × 400 g tin red kidney beans, drained and rinsed
1 tablespoon chopped coriander, plus extra leaves to garnish
salt and freshly ground black pepper
steamed rice, to serve

Heat the canola oil in a large non-stick frying pan over medium–high heat. Add the cumin and chilli powder and cook, stirring, for 1 minute or until fragrant. Add the onion and garlic and cook for about 3 minutes or until the onion has softened.

Reduce the heat to medium–low, add the mince and cook, stirring regularly, for 5–6 minutes or until lightly browned. Stir in the diced tomatoes, tomato paste and kidney beans. Reduce the heat to medium and simmer, stirring occasionally, for 10 minutes or until much of the liquid has evaporated and the mixture has thickened. Remove from the heat, then stir through the coriander and season to taste. Garnish with extra coriander leaves and serve with steamed rice.

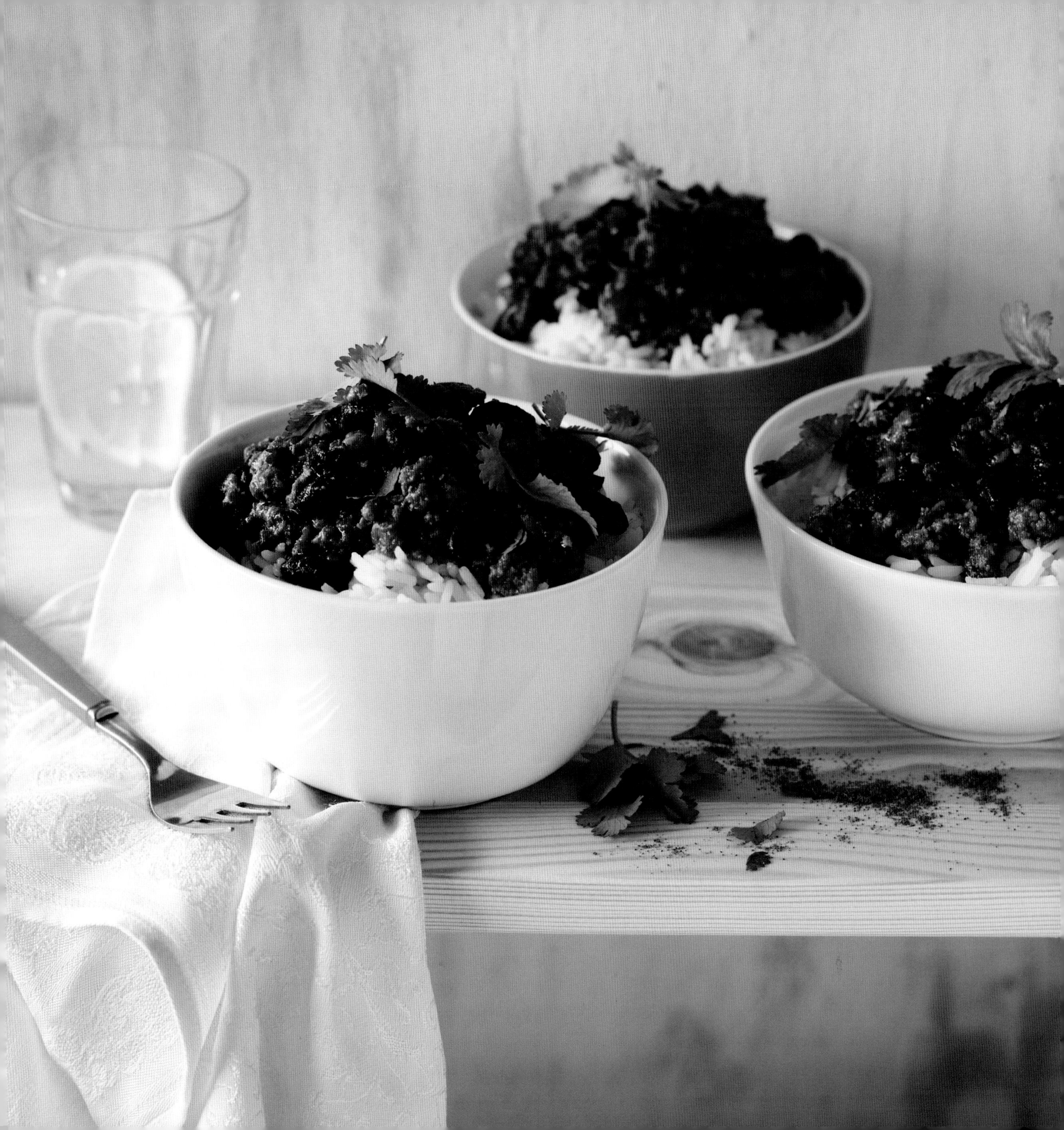

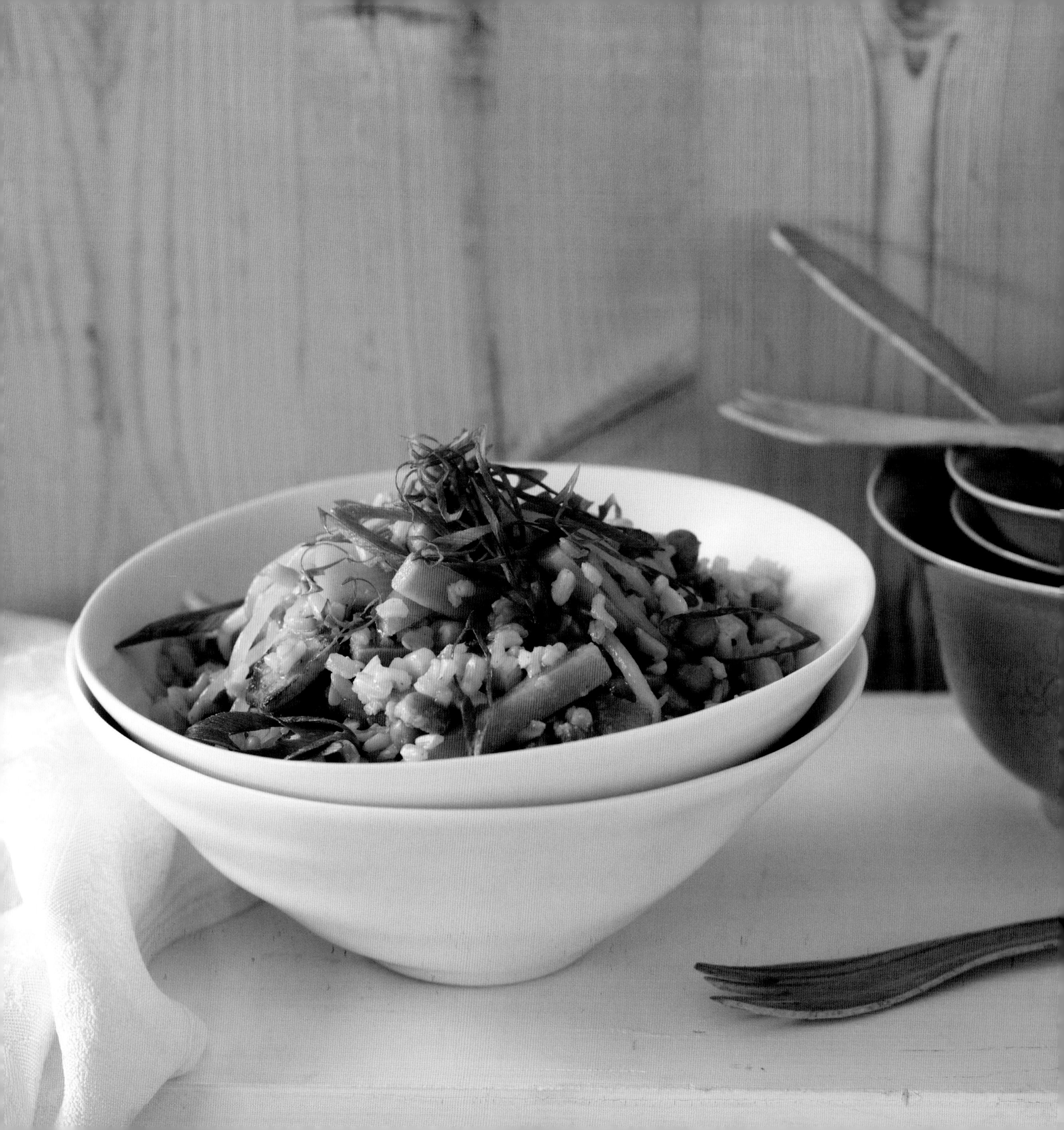

< Fried brown rice

This is a wholegrain, healthier alternative to regular fried rice, which is usually made with white rice. It is also a fabulous way to use up leftover meat, chicken and vegetables. Feel free to substitute your own leftovers for any of the ingredients listed here. SERVES 4

2 litres gluten-free, wheat-free, dairy-free, soy-free chicken stock
2 cups (400 g) long-grain brown rice
2 tablespoons canola oil
3 cloves garlic, crushed
1 tablespoon grated ginger
5 rashers rindless bacon, chopped
1 carrot, cut into matchsticks
¾ cup (90 g) frozen peas
½ cup (100 g) corn kernels
110 g bamboo shoots
1 cup (80 g) bean sprouts
2 spring onions, green part only, thinly sliced on the diagonal
salt and freshly ground black pepper
chopped chilli, to garnish (optional)

Pour the stock into a large saucepan and bring to the boil. Reduce the heat to medium–low, add the rice and cook for about 50 minutes or until the rice is tender, stirring regularly. Drain.

Meanwhile, heat 1 tablespoon canola oil in a large frying pan over medium heat and cook the garlic, ginger and bacon until the bacon is lightly browned. Add the carrot, peas, corn, bamboo shoots and bean sprouts and toss over the heat until the vegetables are tender. Add the rice and stir to combine. Add the remaining canola oil and most of the spring onion and season to taste with salt and pepper. Garnish with chopped chilli, if using, and the remaining spring onion and serve immediately.

Baked beef rendang risotto

Risotto is usually cooked on the stovetop, adding a ladleful of stock at a time. In this recipe, however, you simply put all the ingredients in an ovenproof dish and cook them in the oven. It tastes fantastic and the method is far less time-consuming. If you are allergic to coconut, replace the coconut cream with rice milk. SERVES 4

1 onion, cut into thin wedges
500 g lean beef steak, thinly sliced
1 cup (250 ml) gluten-free, wheat-free, dairy-free, soy-free rendang curry sauce
½ red capsicum (pepper), sliced
1⅓ cups (265 g) arborio rice
1 litre gluten-free, wheat-free, dairy-free, soy-free beef stock
3 tablespoons coconut cream
salad, to serve

Preheat the oven to 150°C.

Place the onion, beef and half the sauce in a 2-litre flameproof casserole dish and cook for 3–4 minutes or until the onion has softened and the beef is lightly browned. Stir in the capsicum, rice and stock.

Transfer the dish to the oven and cook, covered, for 25 minutes. Give it a good stir, then cook for a further hour. Stir in the coconut cream and remaining curry sauce and serve with a salad.

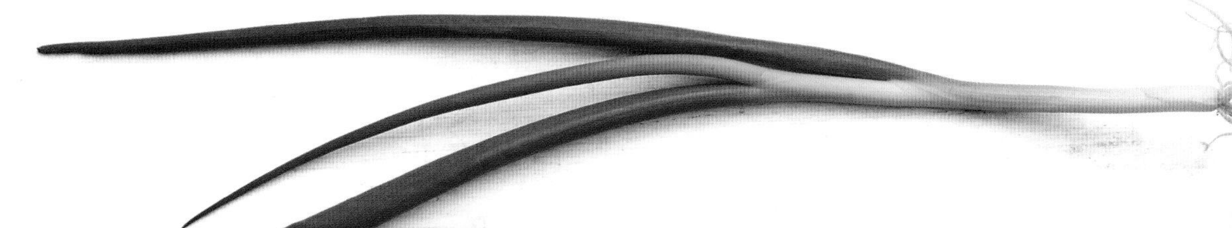

Creole beef with crispy potatoes

Creole cuisine uses plenty of herbs and spices, blending French and Native American ingredients and methods. The seasoning in this recipe also works well with chicken and lamb.

SERVES 4

1 teaspoon onion powder
1 teaspoon garlic powder
1 teaspoon dried basil
½ teaspoon dried thyme
½ teaspoon cayenne pepper
1½ teaspoons paprika
½ teaspoon salt
½ teaspoon freshly ground black pepper
1 tablespoon vegetable oil
4 × 200 g rib-eye steaks
watercress sprigs, to serve

CRISPY POTATOES
20 small new potatoes
⅓ cup (80 ml) olive oil
2 cloves garlic, crushed
juice of 1 lemon
sea salt and freshly ground black pepper

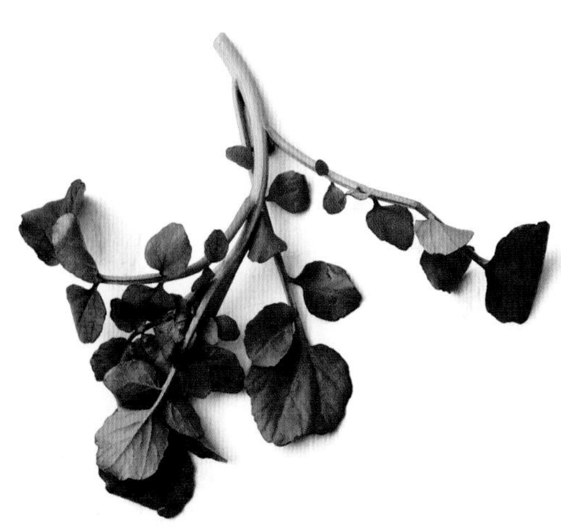

Preheat the oven to 180°C. Grease a large roasting tin.

Place all the dried spices in a small bowl, add the oil and mix well to combine. Brush over both sides of the steaks.

To prepare the crispy potatoes, fill a large saucepan with water and bring to the boil over medium–high heat. Add the potatoes and cook for 5–6 minutes, then drain and set aside.

Combine the olive oil, garlic, lemon, salt and pepper in a small bowl. Use a potato masher to flatten each potato, then place in the roasting tin. Slowly pour the oil mixture over the potatoes, making sure they are evenly coated. Place in the oven and bake for 15 minutes or until golden brown and crispy.

Meanwhile, preheat a grill plate, chargrill pan or barbecue to medium–high and cook the steaks to your liking. Cover and leave to rest for a few minutes.

Serve the steaks with the crispy potatoes and watercress sprigs.

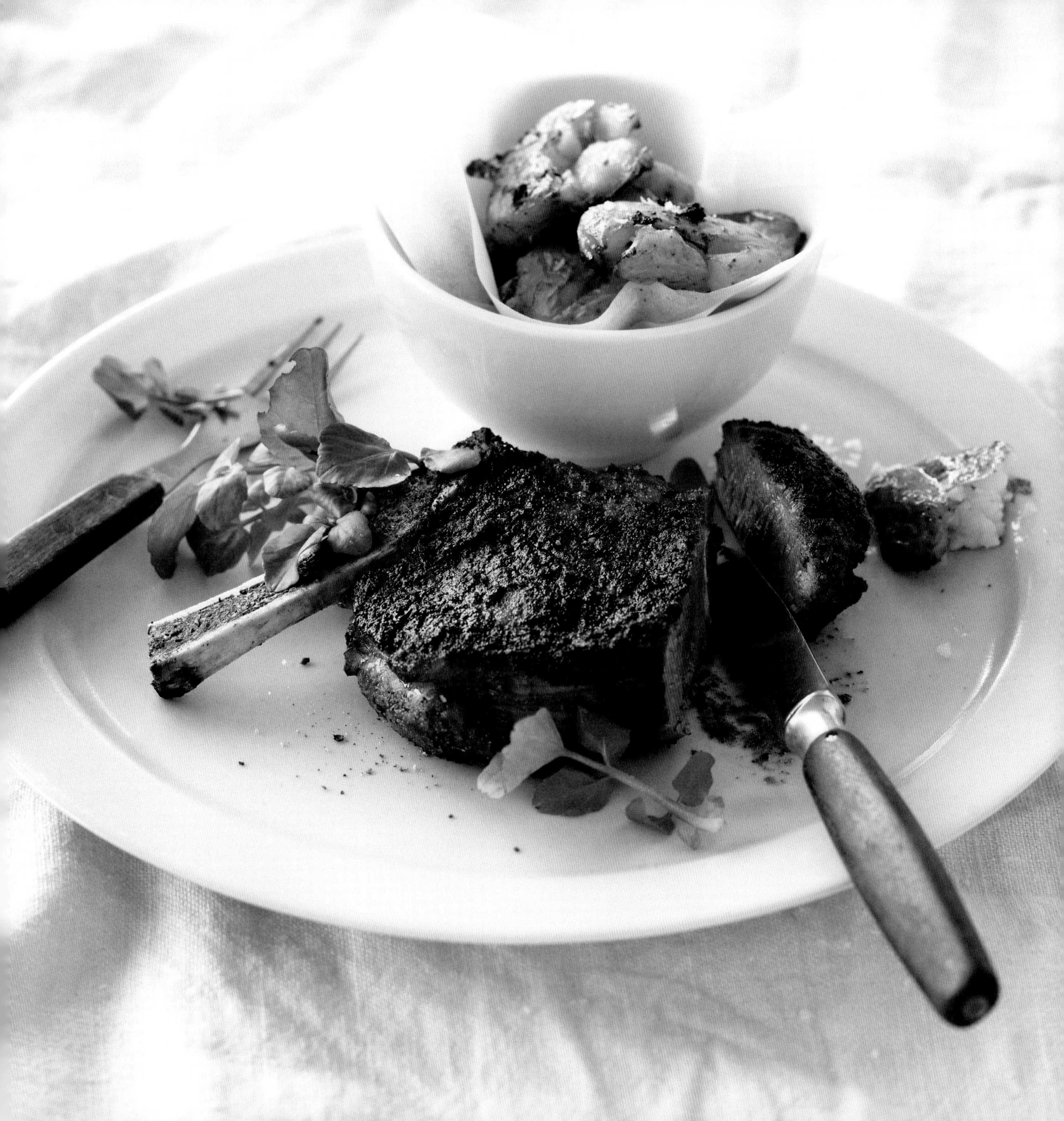

Veal with chunky tomato and olive sauce

Tomatoes, olives and fresh herbs give this dish a distinctly Mediterranean flavour. I love it with veal, but it is also good made with chicken fillets or tuna steaks.

SERVES 4

2 cloves garlic, crushed
1 small onion, finely chopped
1 × 400 g tin crushed tomatoes, drained
2 teaspoons sugar
½ cup (80 g) sliced black olives
2 tablespoons chopped flat-leaf parsley
2 tablespoons chopped oregano
salt and freshly ground black pepper
olive oil, for pan-frying
4 × 150 g veal steaks
steamed green beans, to serve

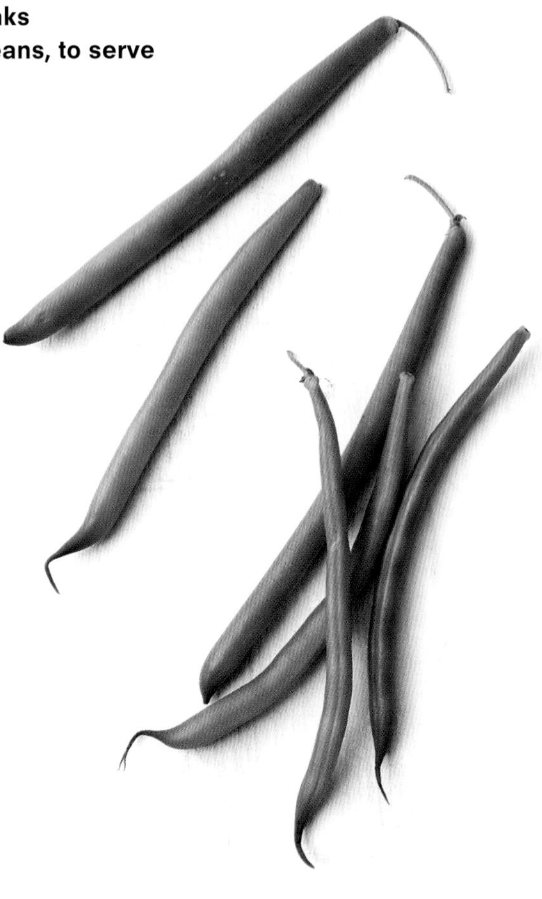

Combine the garlic, onion, crushed tomatoes, sugar and olives in a small frying pan and cook over medium–low heat, stirring occasionally, for 15 minutes. Remove from the heat and stir in the fresh herbs. Season to taste with salt and pepper.

Meanwhile, heat a little olive oil in a large frying pan over medium–high heat. Add the veal steaks and cook for 4–5 minutes each side or until golden brown.

Place a veal steak on each serving plate and spoon over the sauce. Serve with steamed green beans, or your choice of vegetables.

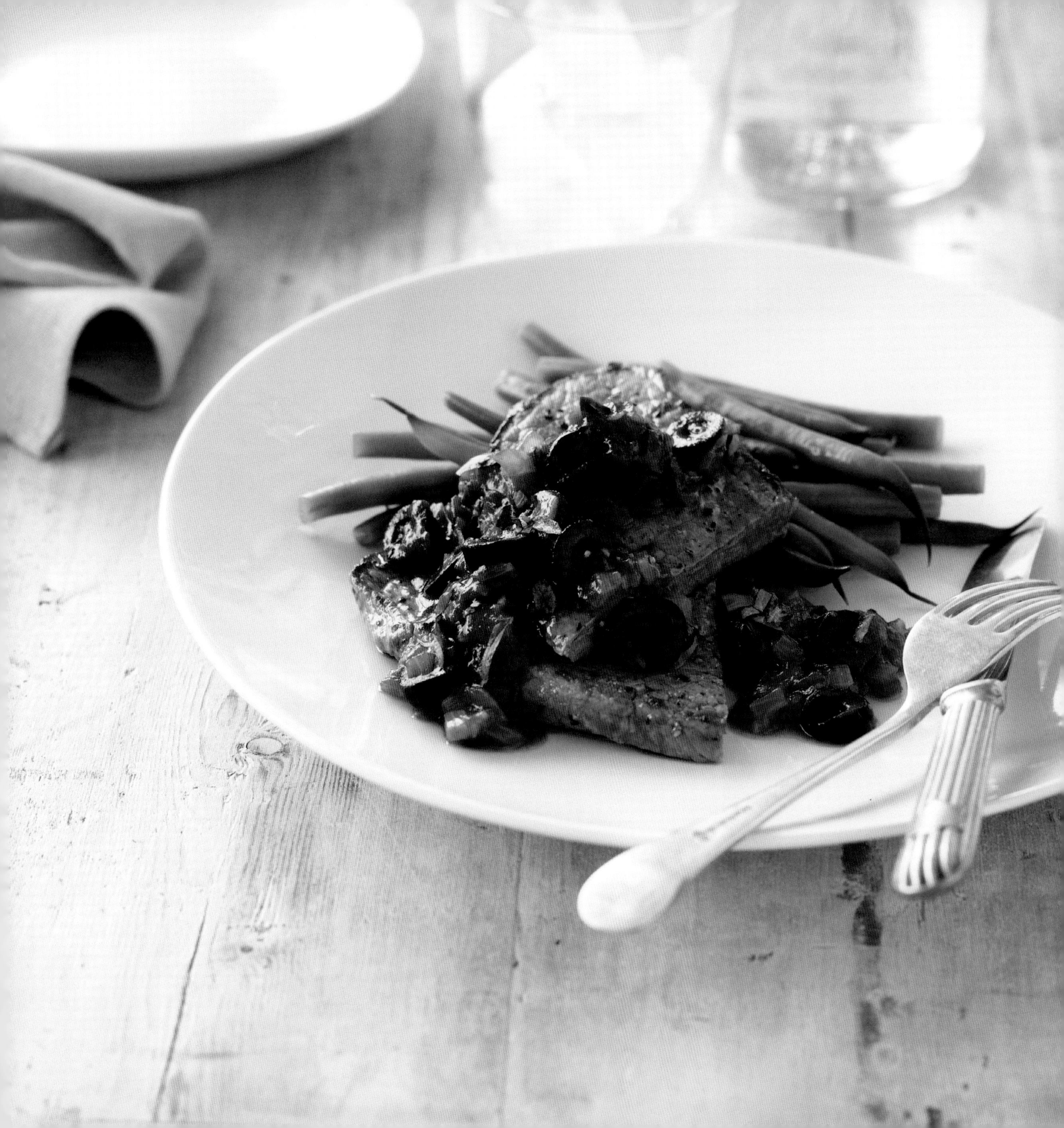

Lamb shanks with garlic and rosemary polenta

'Frenched' lamb shanks have been trimmed and had their fat removed, and are generally more expensive than regular lamb shanks. If they are not available, this recipe works just as well with untrimmed lamb shanks. SERVES 4

8 small or 4 large frenched lamb shanks
1 tablespoon olive oil
1 tablespoon lemon juice
2 cloves garlic, crushed
2 sprigs of rosemary, plus extra leaves to garnish
salt and freshly ground black pepper
1 cup (250 ml) gluten-free, wheat-free, dairy-free, soy-free beef stock
1 teaspoon maize cornflour
steamed greens, to serve

GARLIC AND ROSEMARY POLENTA
3 cups (750 ml) rice milk
2 sprigs of rosemary
2 cloves garlic, lightly crushed
⅔ cup (110 g) instant polenta
salt and freshly ground black pepper

Combine the lamb shanks, olive oil, lemon juice, garlic, rosemary, salt and pepper in a non-metallic bowl and turn to coat. Cover and marinate in the fridge for at least 3 hours.

Preheat the oven to 170°C.

Place the lamb shanks in a baking dish, pour over the stock and cook in the oven for 1½ hours or until tender.

Meanwhile, to prepare the polenta, heat the rice milk, rosemary and garlic in a medium saucepan over medium–high heat until almost boiling. Remove the garlic and rosemary sprigs and reserve for later. Add the polenta and stir until the mixture boils. Reduce the heat to low, then cook, stirring constantly, for further 4–5 minutes or until the polenta is the texture of smooth mashed potato. Season to taste with salt and pepper.

Remove the lamb shanks from oven. Pour the cooking juices into a small frying pan, then cover the shanks with foil and keep warm in a very low oven while you make the sauce.

Combine the cornflour and ½ cup (125 ml) water in a small bowl to form a smooth paste. Place the pan with the cooking juices over medium–low heat and gradually stir in the cornflour paste. Add the reserved garlic and leaves from half a sprig of rosemary and stir until well combined and heated through.

Spoon the polenta onto warmed plates. Top with the lamb shanks, then pour over the sauce. Season with salt and pepper and garnish with the extra rosemary leaves. Serve with your choice of steamed greens.

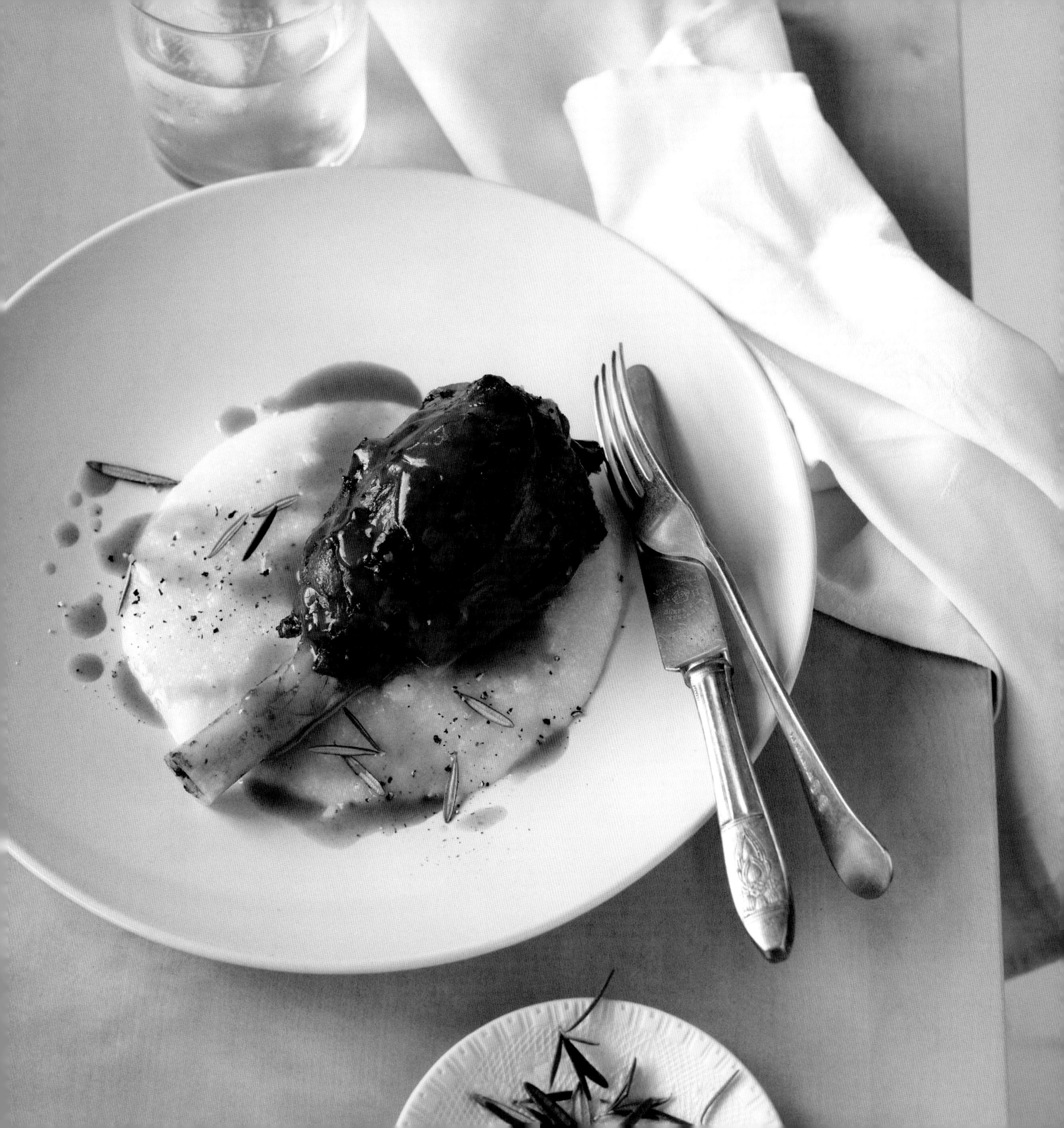

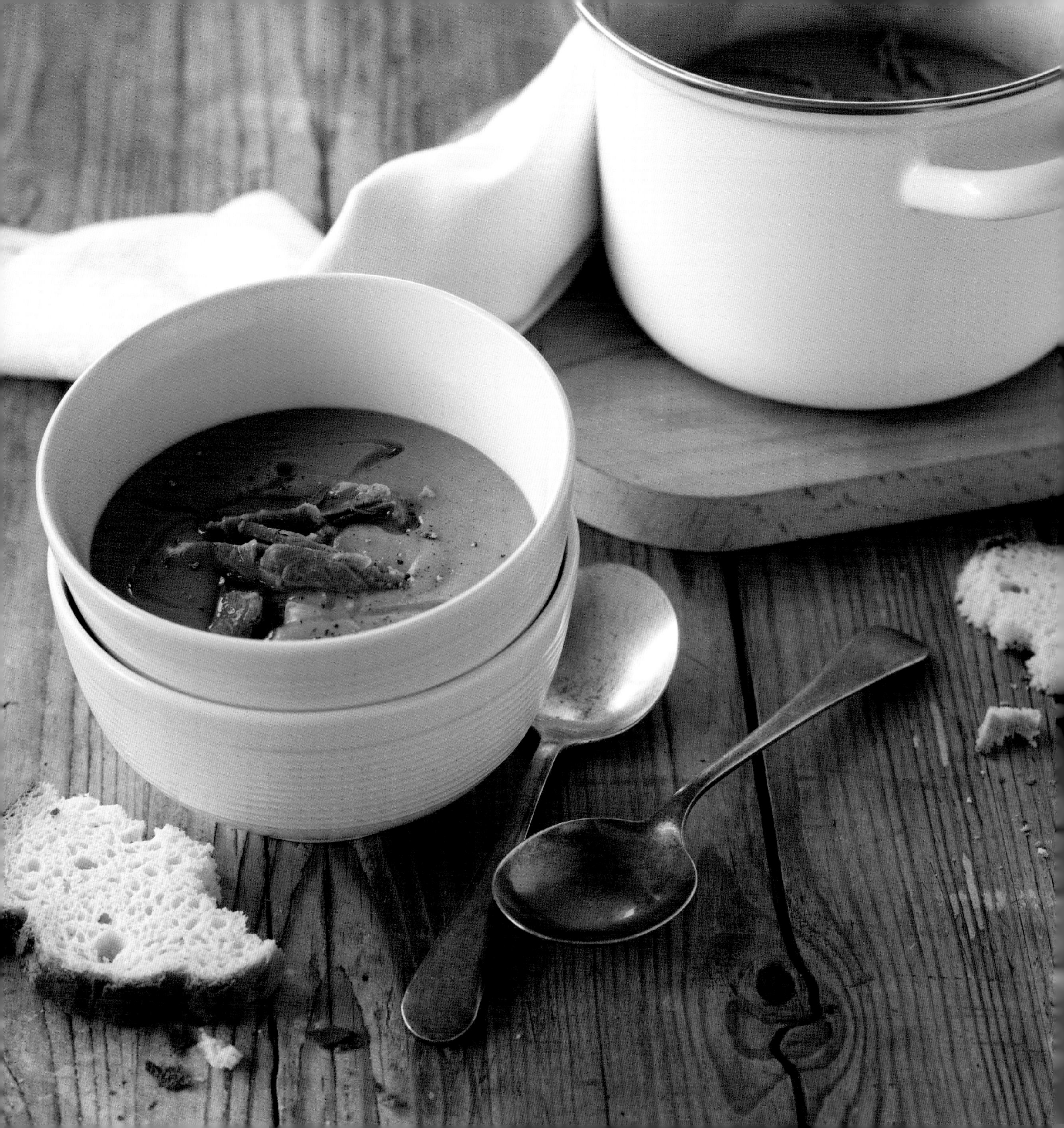

Pea and ham soup

This recipe is an old favourite. Like many soups, it takes a while to cook but it's worth the wait. The smoky flavour of the ham hock permeates the soup and is the perfect complement to the earthiness of the peas. SERVES 4–6

2 teaspoons olive oil
2 carrots, diced
2 potatoes, diced
1 large ham hock
500 g dried green split peas
2 litres gluten-free, wheat-free, dairy-free, soy-free chicken stock
freshly ground black pepper
extra virgin olive oil, for drizzling
gluten-free, wheat-free, dairy-free, soy-free bread, to serve

Heat the olive oil in a large stockpot over medium–high heat. Add the carrot and potato and cook until golden brown. Add the ham hock, split peas and stock, then reduce the heat to low and cook gently for 1 hour, stirring occasionally.

Turn off the heat and take out the ham hock. Allow to cool slightly, then remove the meat from the bone, cutting it into small chunks.

Puree the soup using a blender or hand-held blender, then warm over medium heat. Stir through the ham pieces (reserving a few for garnish, if liked). As soon as the soup starts to simmer, turn off the heat and ladle it into deep bowls. Finish with a grinding of pepper and a drizzle of extra virgin olive oil, then serve with gluten-free, wheat-free, dairy-free, soy-free bread.

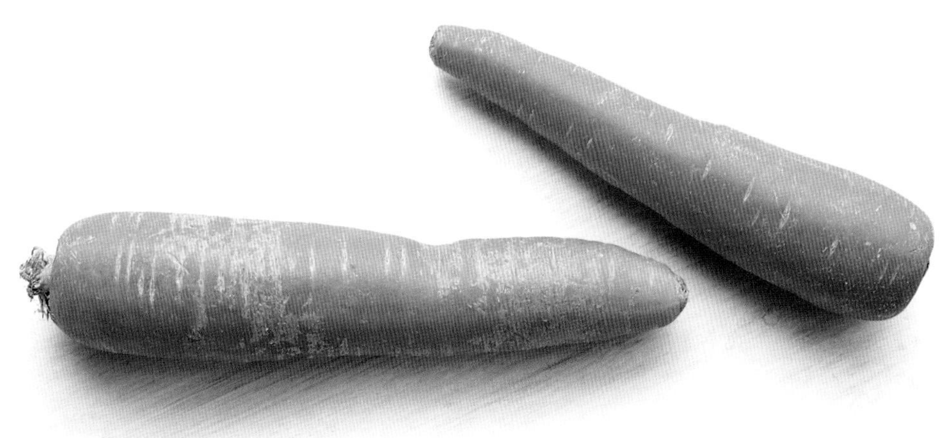

Baked potatoes with chilli beef and bacon

These potatoes make a substantial lunch or a relaxed Sunday-night dinner. The cheese topping is optional – if you are allergic to dairy products, leave it out. SERVES 4

4 large potatoes, unpeeled
2 teaspoons olive oil
2 cloves garlic, crushed
1 onion, chopped
5 rashers rindless bacon, diced
400 g lean minced beef
½–1 teaspoon chilli powder
1 carrot, grated
2 cups (500 ml) pureed tomato
salt and freshly ground black pepper
soy-free, dairy-free spread, to serve
grated cheddar, to serve (optional)

Preheat the oven to 180°C.

Place the potatoes on a baking tray and bake for 1 hour. Turn the heat off and leave them in the oven to stay warm while you make the filling.

Heat the olive oil in a large non-stick frying pan over medium heat. Add the garlic, onion and bacon and cook until the onion is soft and the bacon is crispy. Add the minced beef, chilli powder, carrot and pureed tomato. Reduce the heat to medium–low and simmer for about 10 minutes, stirring occasionally. Season to taste.

Remove the potatoes from the oven. Place in a shallow bowl and cut into thick wedges. Dob a little dairy-free spread over the potato and allow it to melt, then spoon the warm filling over the top. Sprinkle with grated cheddar (if using) and serve.

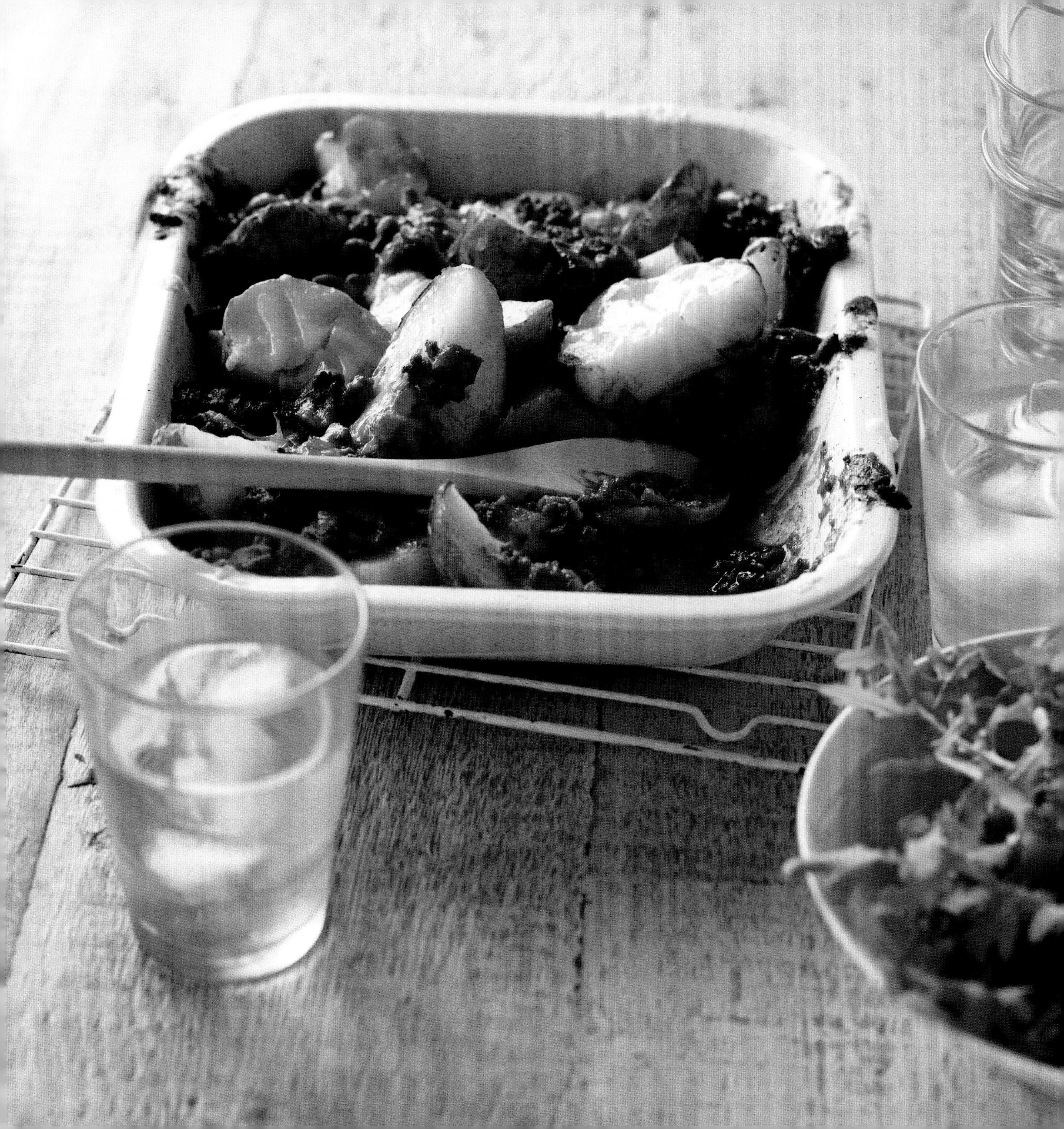

Beef in plum sauce

This recipe includes a little soy sauce. If you're allergic to soy, leave it out or use molasses and apple cider vinegar, as described in the note at the end. SERVES 4

1 tablespoon vegetable oil
1 clove garlic, crushed
1 teaspoon Chinese five-spice powder
½ teaspoon ground ginger
½ teaspoon paprika
600 g stir-fry beef strips
1 carrot, cut into thin slices on the diagonal
2 sticks celery, cut into thin slices on the diagonal
425 g tin baby corn, drained
100 g green beans, trimmed if liked
½ cup (125 ml) strong gluten-free, wheat-free, dairy-free, soy-free beef stock
1 teaspoon gluten-free, wheat-free soy sauce* (optional)
1½ tablespoons maize cornflour
¾ cup (240 g) plum jam
salt and freshly ground black pepper
coriander leaves, to garnish
steamed rice, to serve

Heat the vegetable oil in a large saucepan over medium heat. Add the garlic and spices and cook for 1 minute or until fragrant. Add the beef and cook for 3–4 minutes, stirring regularly to brown well. Add the vegetables, stock and soy sauce (if using), then cover and simmer for 4–6 minutes or until the vegetables are tender.

In a small bowl, blend the cornflour with 3 tablespoons water to make a paste. Add the plum jam and stir well to combine. Add to the pan and stir through the meat and vegetables until thickened. Garnish with coriander leaves and serve with steamed rice.

***For soy allergy**
In a small bowl, combine ¾ teaspoon molasses and ¼ teaspoon apple cider vinegar. Use in place of the soy sauce.

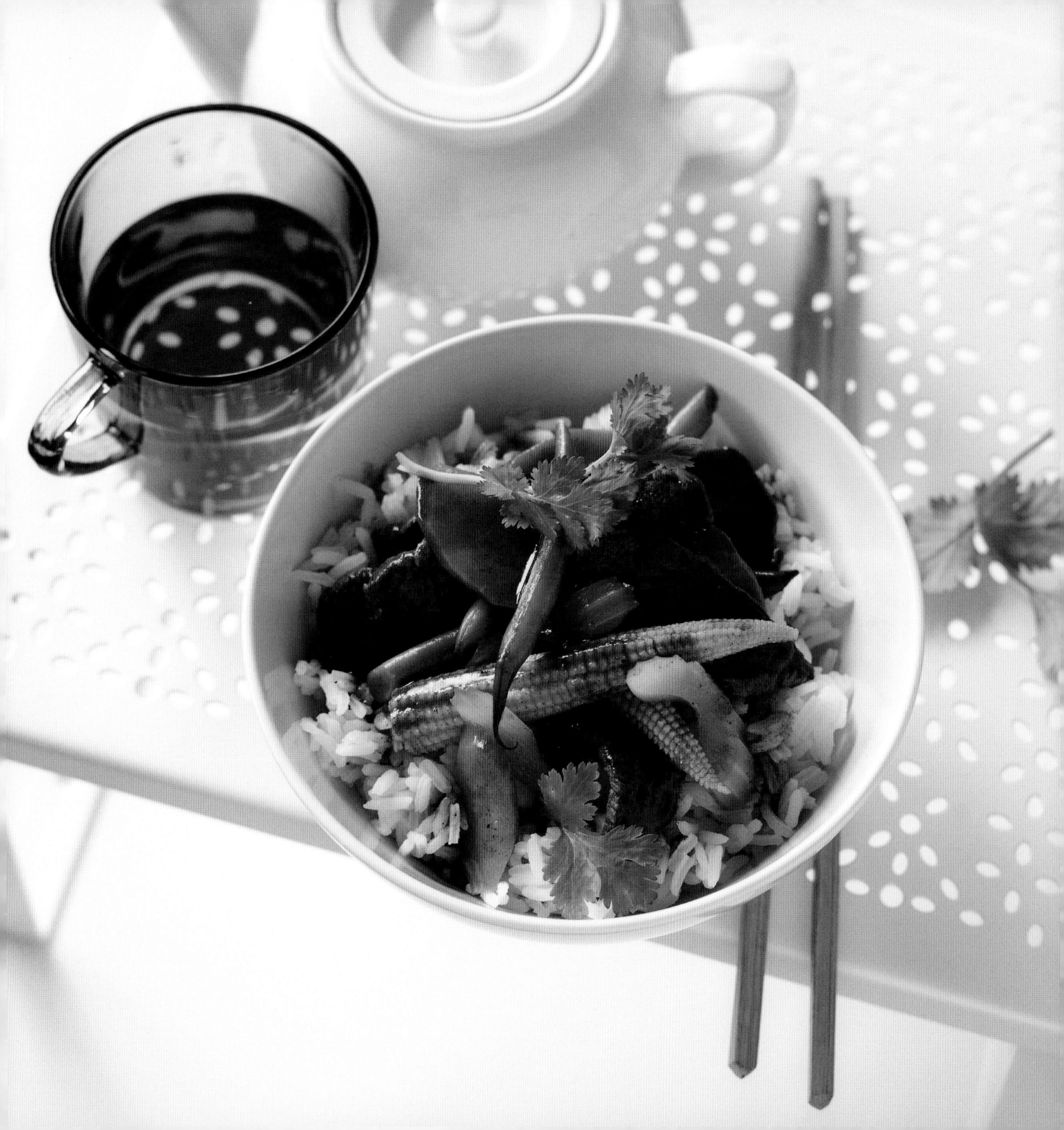

Garlic pepper lamb stir-fry

A wok is the classic piece of equipment for cooking Asian stir-fries, but if you don't own one a large non-stick frying pan is a good substitute. SERVES 4

1 tablespoon canola oil
4 cloves garlic, crushed
1 teaspoon grated ginger
400 g lamb steak, thinly sliced
1 cup (250 ml) gluten-free, wheat-free, dairy-free, soy-free beef stock
1 tablespoon maize cornflour
1 tablespoon gluten-free, wheat-free soy sauce*
freshly ground black pepper, to taste
1 small head broccoli, cut into florets
2 cups (200 g) snowpeas (mange-tout), trimmed and halved on the diagonal
1 cup (80 g) bean sprouts, rinsed
1 carrot, cut into matchsticks
salt and freshly ground black pepper
rice noodles or steamed rice, to serve

Heat the canola oil in a large wok or frying pan over medium–high heat. Add the garlic and ginger and cook for 1 minute or until fragrant. Add the lamb strips and cook until lightly browned on all sides.

In a small bowl, blend a little stock with the cornflour to make a paste. Add the remaining stock and soy sauce and stir until smooth. Season with pepper.

Add the broccoli, snowpeas, bean sprouts and carrot to the wok or pan and stir-fry for 2–4 minutes or until just tender. Pour in the sauce and cook for 1–2 minutes or until thickened slightly and coating the meat and vegetables. Taste, and add more salt and pepper if needed. Serve immediately over rice noodles or steamed rice.

***For soy allergy**
In a small bowl, combine 3 teaspoons molasses and 1 teaspoon apple cider vinegar. Use in place of the soy sauce.

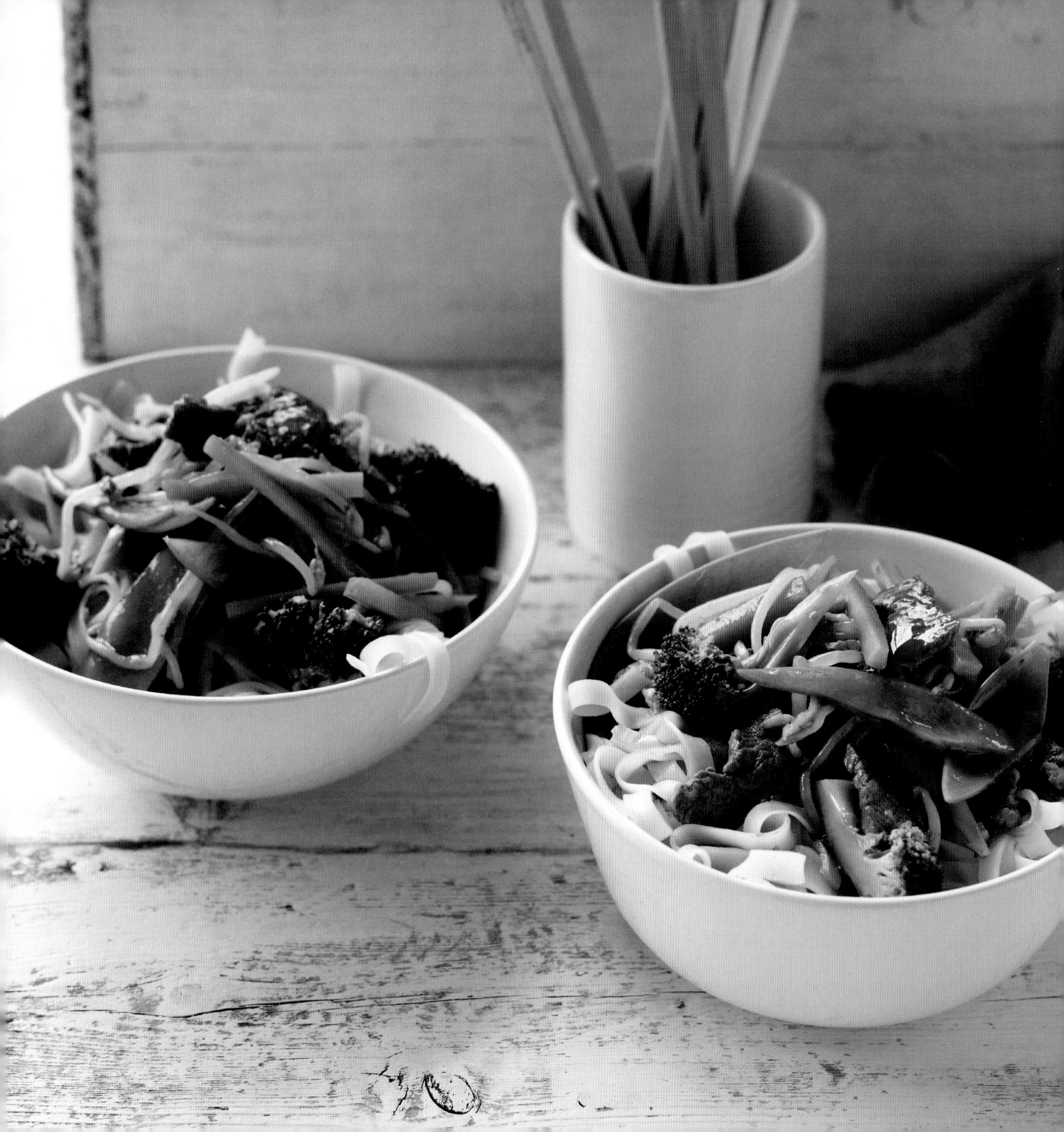

Osso buco

Osso buco means 'bone with a hole' in Italian. It is a cut of veal shank with the bone in, and the 'hole' is left after you've eaten the marrow in the centre. The tender meat falls away from the bone in this dish in a very appealing way, and the marrow is a real delicacy. SERVES 4

⅓ cup (50 g) maize cornflour
salt and freshly ground black pepper
8 × 250 g pieces osso buco
⅓ cup (80 ml) olive oil
1 onion, diced
3 small carrots, diced
120 g button mushrooms, sliced
3 sticks celery, sliced
2 cloves garlic, crushed
1 teaspoon dried chilli flakes (or to taste)
3 cups (750 ml) gluten-free, wheat-free, dairy-free, soy-free beef stock
1½ cups (375 ml) pureed tomato
3 tablespoons chopped flat-leaf parsley, plus extra to garnish
1 tablespoon dried Italian herbs
1 tablespoon chopped oregano
mashed potato, rice or garlic and rosemary polenta (see page 64), to serve

In a shallow bowl, combine the cornflour, salt and pepper. Toss each piece of meat in the flour mixture, shaking off any excess.

Heat 2 tablespoons olive oil in a large stockpot or flameproof casserole dish. Add half the osso buco and cook for 2–3 minutes or until browned on both sides. Remove and repeat with the remaining olive oil and osso buco. Remove the meat pieces and set aside.

Add the onion, carrot, mushroom, celery, garlic and chilli to the pan and toss through the meat cooking juices. Return the osso buco, then add the stock, pureed tomato and herbs and stir until well combined. Reduce the heat and simmer for 40–50 minutes, stirring occasionally, until the meat is tender and the sauce has reduced and thickened. Garnish with extra parsley and serve immediately with mashed potato, rice or polenta.

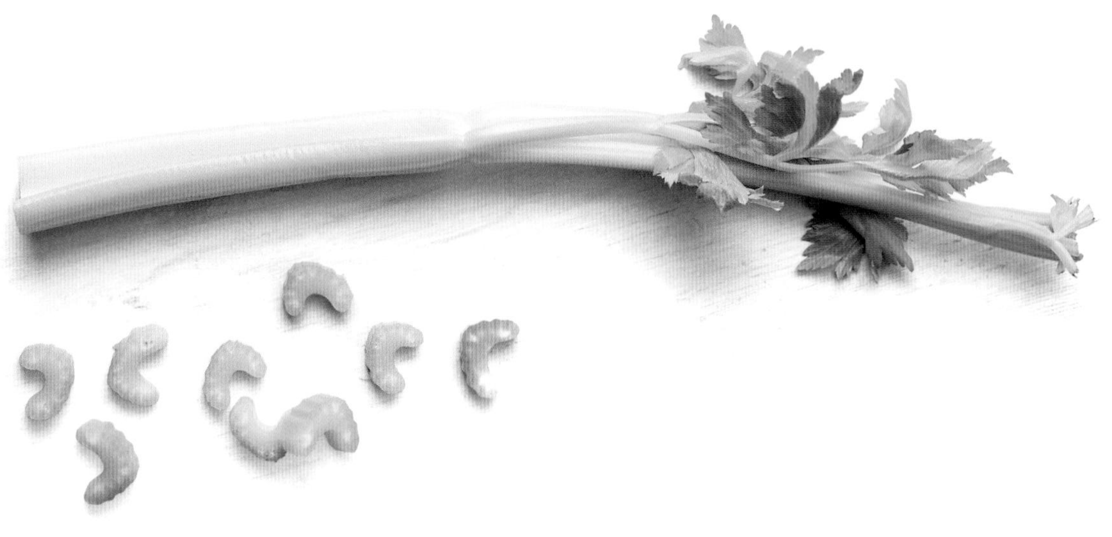

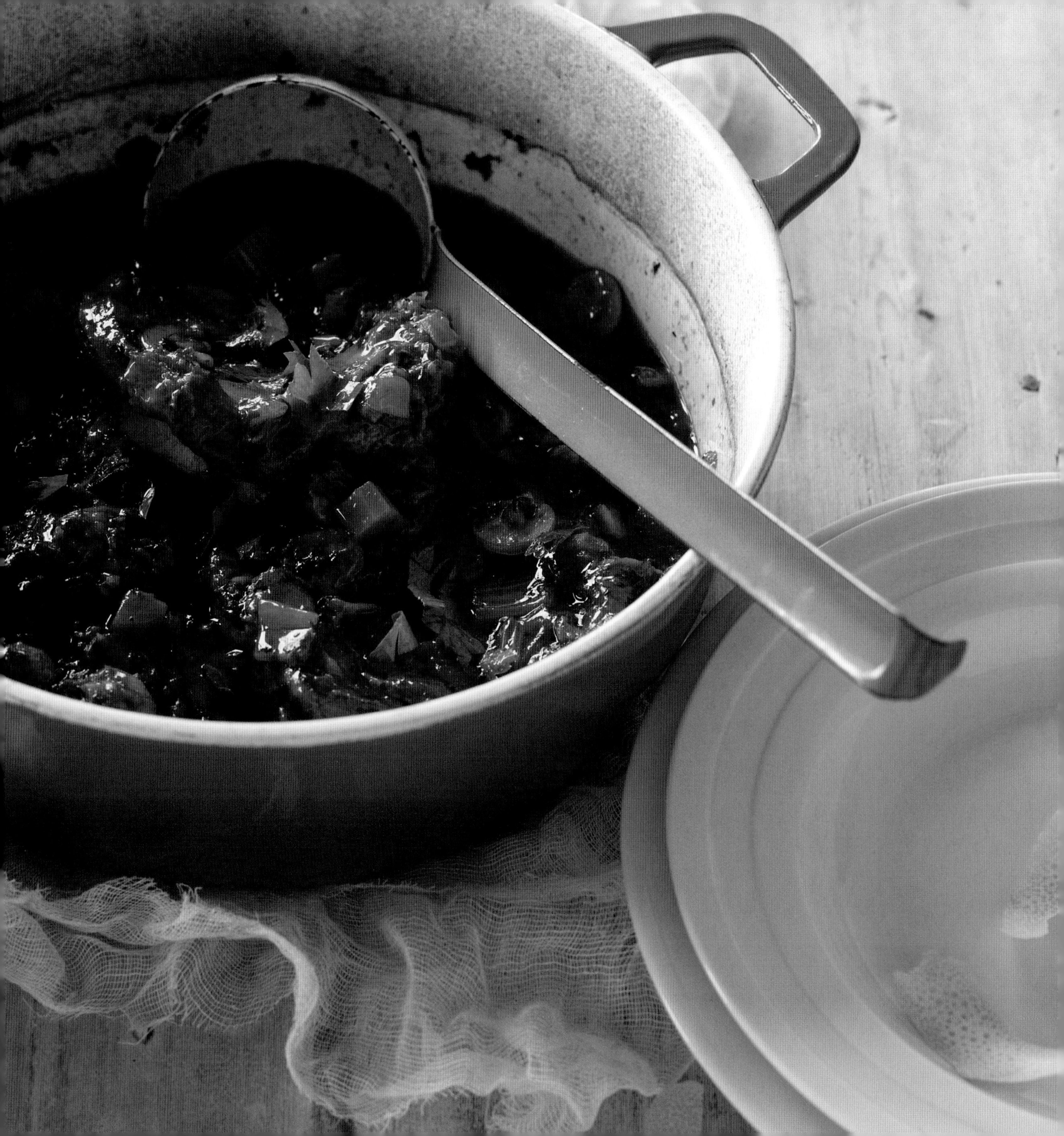

Chow mein

This terrific, messy mix of ingredients makes a popular family meal. The flavour of minced pork works particularly well here, but you could use beef or lamb mince instead if you prefer.

SERVES 4

1 tablespoon canola oil
3 cups (240 g) finely chopped savoy cabbage
4 sticks celery, sliced
2 carrots, diced
100 g tinned bamboo shoots, drained
2 cloves garlic, crushed
1 tablespoon grated ginger
1 tablespoon gluten-free, wheat-free, dairy-free, soy-free curry powder
500 g lean minced pork
2 tablespoons maize cornflour
2 cups (500 ml) gluten-free, wheat-free, dairy-free, soy-free beef stock
1 tablespoon gluten-free, wheat-free soy sauce*
100 g gluten-free rice vermicelli noodles

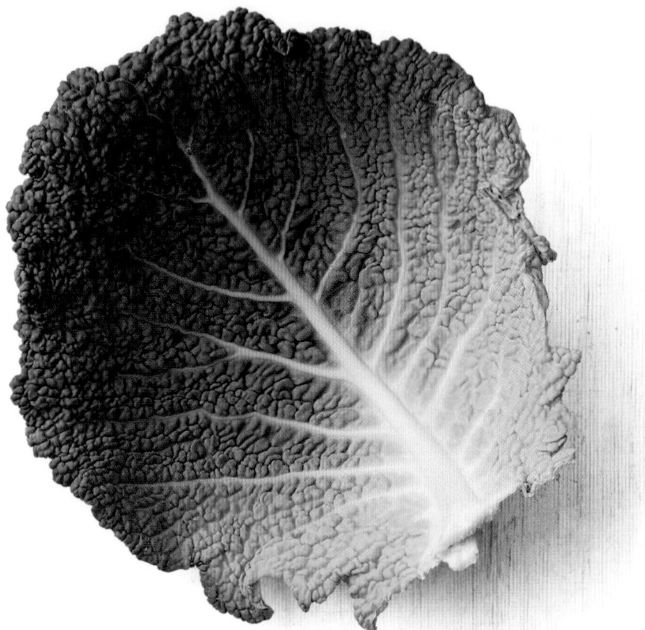

Heat 2 teaspoons canola oil in a large non-stick frying pan, add the cabbage, celery, carrot and bamboo shoots and stir-fry until tender. Remove to a plate.

Heat the remaining oil in the same pan over medium heat, add the garlic, ginger and curry powder and stir for a minute or until fragrant. Add the minced pork and cook until just browned, breaking up any lumps as you go.

In a small bowl, mix together the cornflour, stock and soy sauce until smooth. Add to the pan with the cooked vegetables and stir through until well combined and the sauce has thickened. Reduce the heat to low and simmer for 15–20 minutes, stirring regularly to prevent the mixture sticking to the pan.

Meanwhile, break the rice noodles into short lengths (if liked), place in a bowl and cover with boiling water. Soak for 10 minutes or until softened. Drain. Stir through the pork and vegetable mixture and serve.

***For soy allergy**
In a small bowl, combine 3 teaspoons molasses and 1 teaspoon apple cider vinegar. Use in place of the soy sauce.

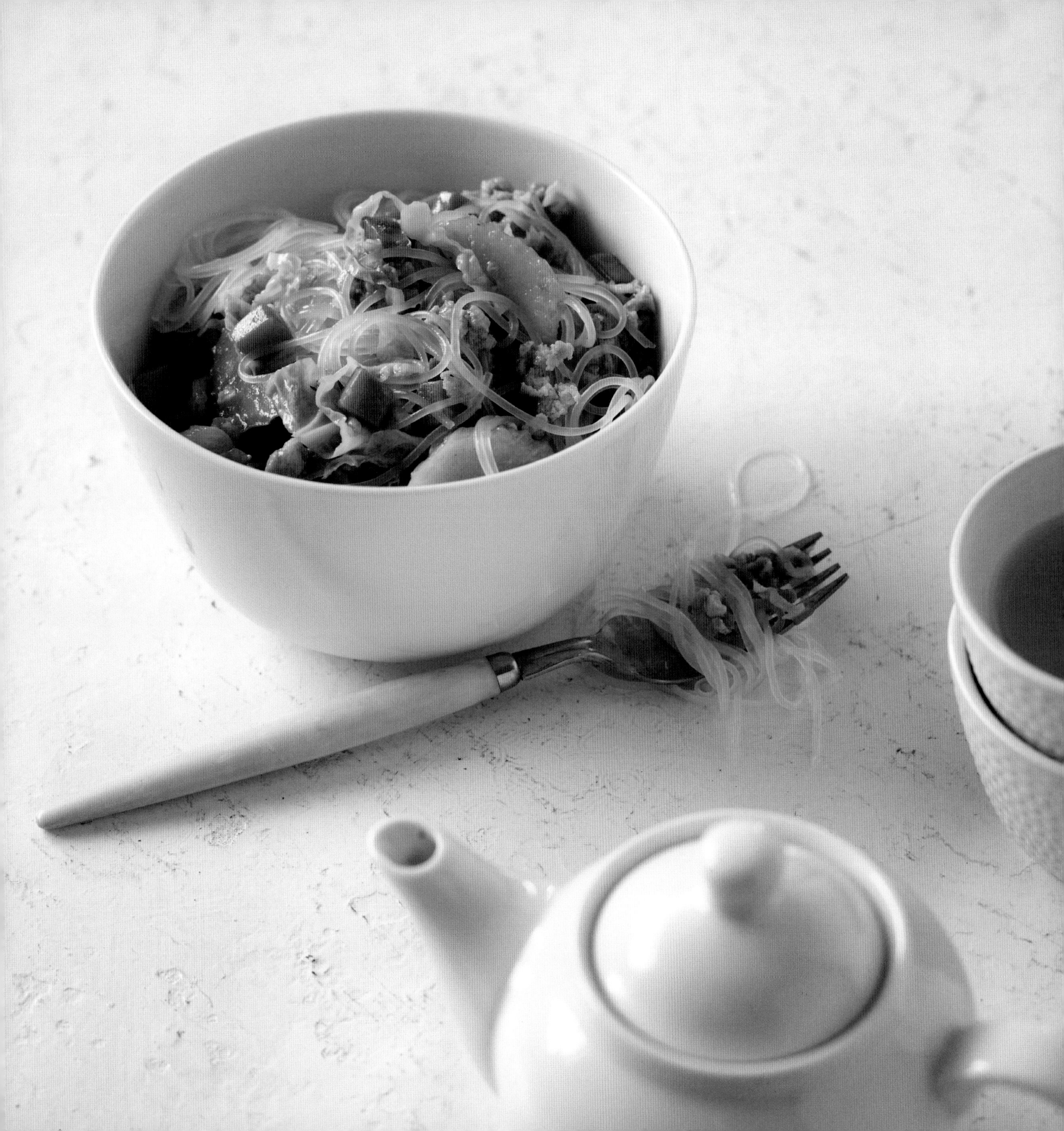

Roast pork cutlets with citrus glaze

This sharpness of this citrus glaze is a perfect foil to the fatty sweetness of the pork cutlets. It would also taste delicious with chicken breast fillets or chicken skewers. I often serve this with the citrus fennel salad on page 18.

SERVES 4

2 cloves garlic, crushed
1 teaspoon celery salt
¼ teaspoon mustard powder
⅓ cup (115 g) orange marmalade
1 tablespoon grated orange zest
juice of 1 orange
freshly ground black pepper
1 tablespoon olive oil
4 × 180 g pork loin cutlets
1 orange, thinly sliced
salad or vegetables, to serve

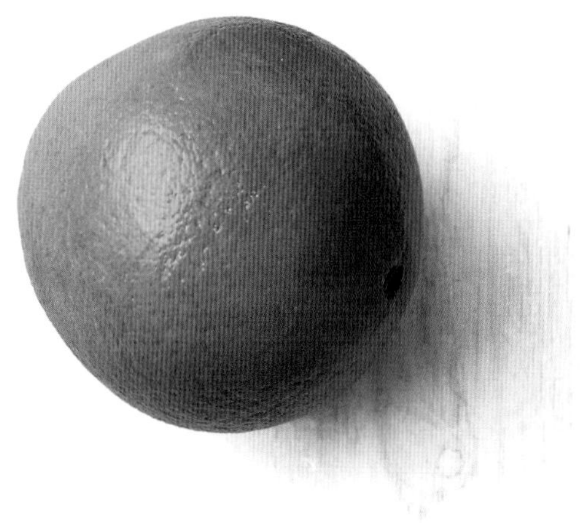

Place the garlic, celery salt, mustard powder, marmalade, orange zest, orange juice, pepper and olive oil in a bowl and combine well. Brush over the pork, then cover and marinate in the fridge for 2–3 hours.

Preheat the oven to 180°C.

Place the pork chops and orange slices in a baking dish or roasting tin and cover with foil. Bake for 10 minutes, then remove the foil and bake for a further 10–15 minutes or until the pork is cooked through. Serve with your choice of salad or vegetables.

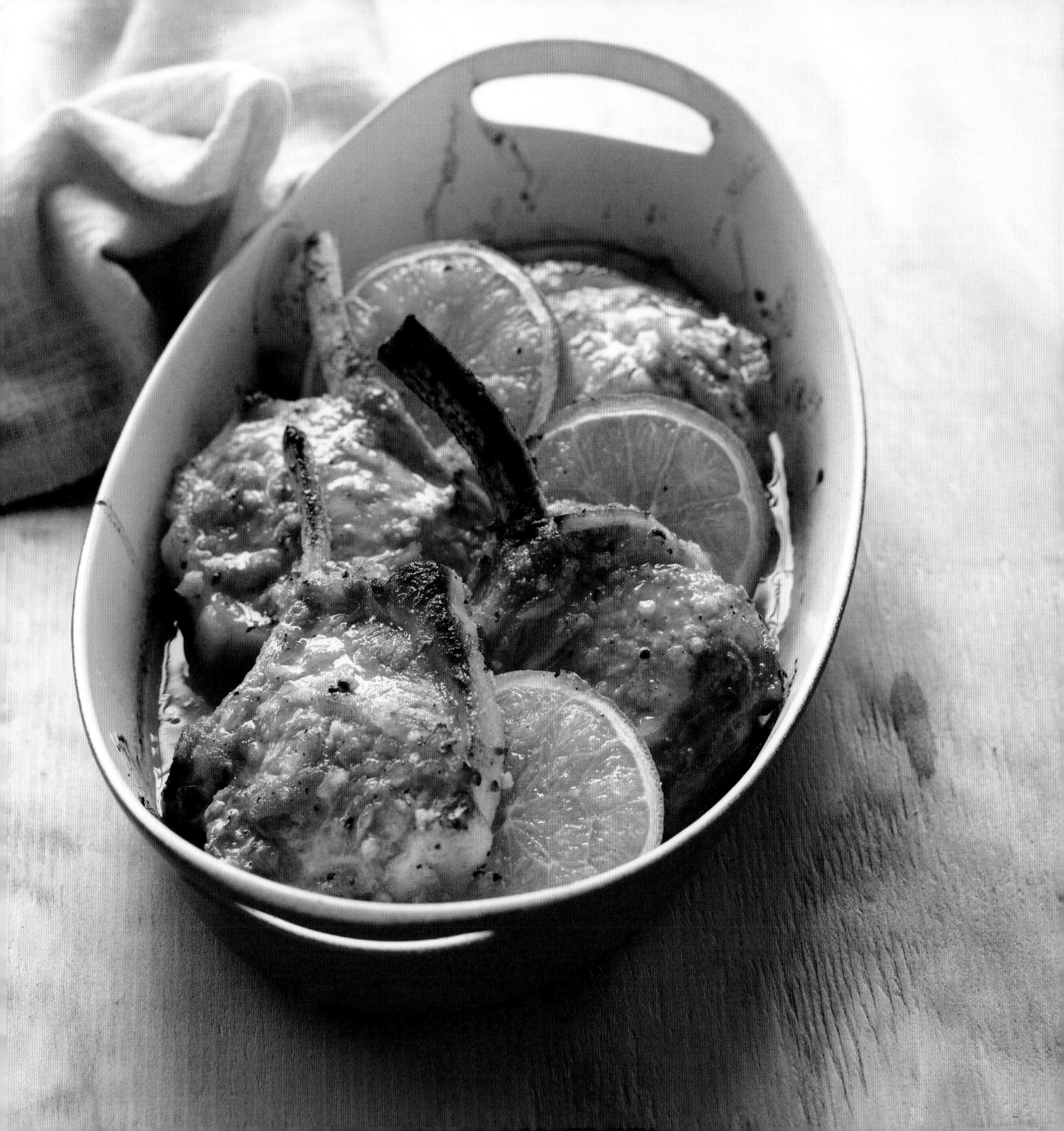

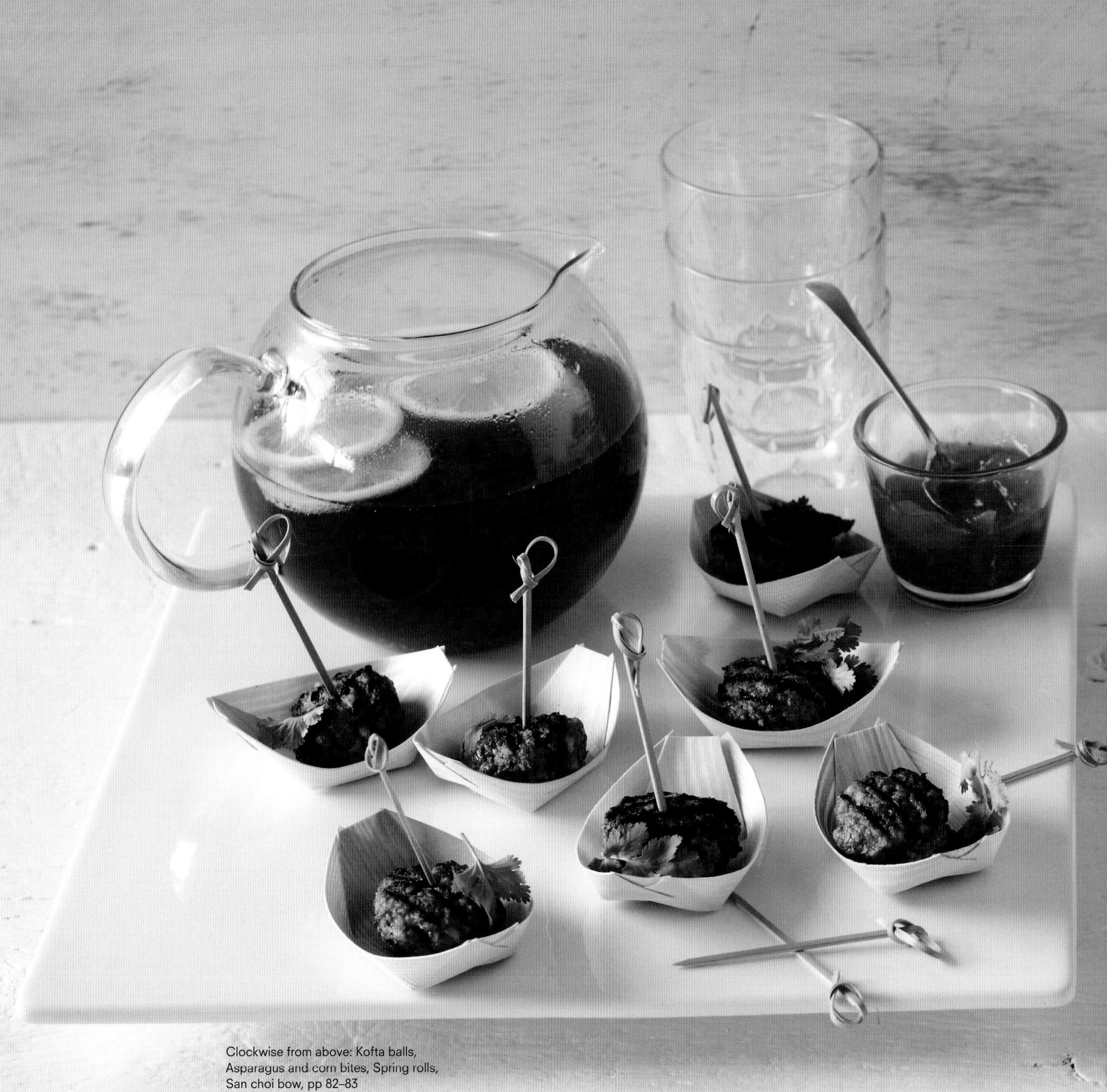

Clockwise from above: Kofta balls, Asparagus and corn bites, Spring rolls, San choi bow, pp 82–83

finger food

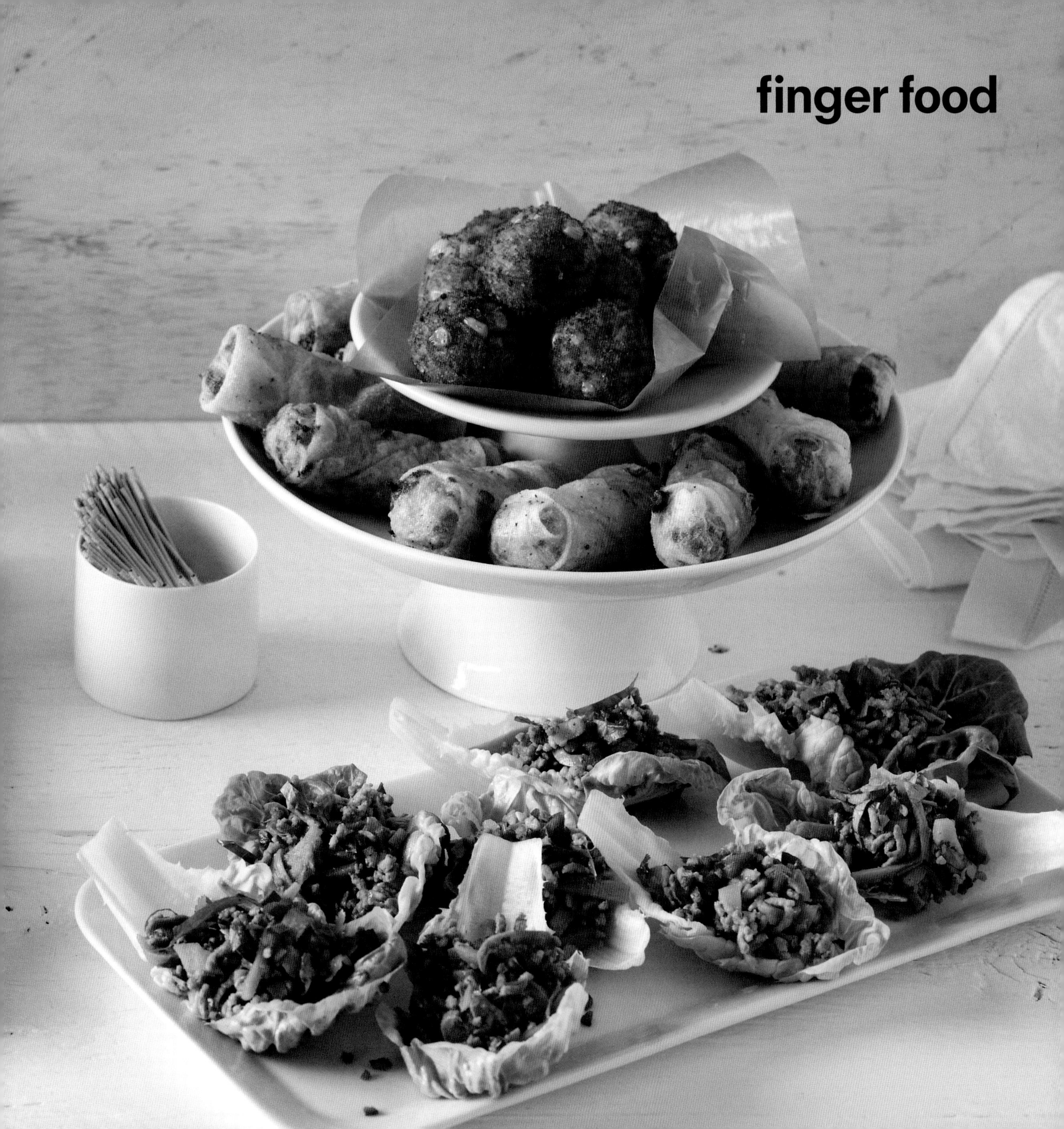

Spring rolls

Although these rolls may seem fiddly to make at first, persevere as I promise they will become easier.

MAKES 24

1 tablespoon cooking sherry
1½ tablespoons gluten-free, wheat-free soy sauce*
1 teaspoon canola oil
3 cloves garlic, crushed
1 tablespoon grated ginger
1 gluten-free, wheat-free, dairy-free, soy-free beef stock cube, crumbled
1 tablespoon maize cornflour
350 g lean minced pork
350 g lean minced beef
⅔ cup (130 g) finely chopped bamboo shoots
½ carrot, finely grated
1 cup (80 g) finely chopped savoy or Chinese cabbage
1 egg, lightly beaten**
24 × 16 cm round rice paper sheets
canola or sunflower oil, for deep-frying
gluten-free, wheat-free sweet chilli sauce, for dipping

Preheat the oven to 150°C.

In a small bowl, mix together the sherry, soy sauce, canola oil, garlic, ginger, stock cube and cornflour.

Combine the minced pork, minced beef, bamboo shoots, carrot and cabbage in a large bowl. Add the garlic mixture and mix together well. Add the egg and mix again.

Fill a large flan dish with hot water. Place a rice paper sheet in the water and soak until softened. Remove from the water and blot dry on paper towel or a clean tea towel. Place 1½ tablespoons of the filling in a line about 4 cm long on the bottom third of the rice paper sheet. Roll the sheet over once, then fold in the edges and continue to roll up tightly like a cigar. Set aside on a plate, seam-side down, and repeat with the remaining rice paper sheets and filling.

Pour the canola or sunflower oil into a deep heavy-based saucepan and heat to 180°C (a cube of bread dropped in the oil should brown in 15 seconds). Working in small batches, deep-fry the spring rolls for 5–6 minutes or until golden. Remove with a slotted spoon and drain on paper towel. Keep warm in the oven while you make the rest. Serve hot with sweet chilli sauce.

***For soy allergy**
In a bowl, combine 1 tablespoon molasses and 1½ teaspoons apple cider vinegar. Use in place of the soy sauce.

****For egg allergy**
Place 1 teaspoon psyllium husks in a small bowl and pour over 3 tablespoons boiling water, stirring constantly to ensure the psyllium does not clump together. Set aside for 4–5 minutes until it forms a gel, stirring occasionally. Use in place of the egg.

San choi bow

When ordered at a restaurant, this dish is usually not suitable for those with food allergies so I've created a variation for you to enjoy at home.

SERVES 10–12

1 tablespoon canola oil
2 cloves garlic, crushed
2 teaspoons finely grated ginger
500 g lean minced pork
190 g tin champignons, drained and sliced
225 g tin water chestnuts, drained and finely chopped
⅓ cup (65 g) bamboo shoots, finely chopped
1 tablespoon chopped coriander
1 tablespoon lemon juice
1½–2 tablespoons gluten-free, wheat-free sweet chilli sauce
1 tablespoon gluten-free, wheat-free soy sauce*
salt
10–12 baby cos lettuce leaves, rinsed and dried

Heat the canola oil in a wok over medium heat, add the garlic and ginger and stir-fry until golden. Add the pork and stir-fry over high heat for 3–4 minutes or until browned, breaking up any lumps as you go. Drain off any excess juices. Add the champignons, water chestnuts, bamboo shoots, coriander, lemon juice, sweet chilli sauce and soy sauce and stir-fry for 2 minutes.

Spoon the mixture into the lettuce cups using a slotted spoon and serve.

***For soy allergy**
In a bowl, combine 3 teaspoons molasses and 1 teaspoon apple cider vinegar. Use in place of the soy sauce.

Kofta balls

These spicy meatballs are sure to please a hungry crowd. The prepared dipping sauces I've suggested below are available in the Indian section of most supermarkets. If you don't have a dairy allergy, you may also wish to serve them with a yoghurt dip, such as tzatziki. MAKES 15–20

600 g lean minced beef
1 egg, lightly beaten*
⅓ cup (25 g) fresh gluten-free, wheat-free, dairy-free, soy-free breadcrumbs
3 tablespoons chopped flat-leaf parsley
1 teaspoon ground cinnamon
1½ tablespoons ground cumin
½ teaspoon chilli powder (or to taste)
3 teaspoons ground turmeric
1½ teaspoons ground allspice
cooking spray
gluten-free, wheat-free, dairy-free, soy-free eggplant pickle or mango chutney, to serve

Place all the ingredients except the cooking spray and pickle or chutney in a large bowl and mix with your hands until well combined. Shape into walnut-sized balls.

Spray a large non-stick frying pan with cooking spray, add 8–10 balls at a time and cook over medium heat until evenly browned and cooked through.

Serve hot with eggplant pickle or mango chutney for dipping.

***For egg allergy**
Place 1 teaspoon psyllium husks in a small bowl and pour over 3 tablespoons boiling water, stirring constantly to ensure the psyllium does not clump together. Set aside for 4–5 minutes until it forms a gel, stirring occasionally. Use in place of the egg.

Asparagus and corn bites

Glutinous rice is a sticky rice that can be purchased at Asian grocers. And don't be fooled by its name – glutinous rice does not contain gluten! MAKES 30

3 cups (750 ml) strong gluten-free, wheat-free, dairy-free, soy-free vegetable stock
¾ cup (150 g) glutinous rice
210 g tin asparagus, drained and mashed
¾ cup (150 g) corn kernels
1 egg, lightly beaten*
1⅓ cups (135 g) dried gluten-free, wheat-free, dairy-free, soy-free breadcrumbs, plus extra if needed
canola oil, for pan-frying

Heat the stock in a large saucepan, add the rice and cook until tender. Drain any excess liquid and place in a medium bowl. While still warm, stir in the asparagus, corn kernels, egg and ⅓ cup (35 g) breadcrumbs. Mix until well combined, then set aside to cool to room temperature.

Preheat the oven to 150°C.

Roll the rice mixture into balls the size of golf balls (add more breadcrumbs if needed to firm up the mixture). Pour the remaining breadcrumbs into a shallow bowl, then add the rice balls and toss until well coated.

Heat a little canola oil in medium frying pan over medium–high heat. Add about 10 rice balls to the pan and cook, turning often, until evenly browned all over. Transfer to a baking tray and keep warm in the oven while you cook the rest, adding more canola oil as required. Serve warm.

***For egg allergy**
Place 1 teaspoon psyllium husks in a small bowl and pour over 3 tablespoons boiling water, stirring constantly to ensure the psyllium does not clump together. Set aside for 4–5 minutes until it forms a gel, stirring occasionally. Use in place of the egg.

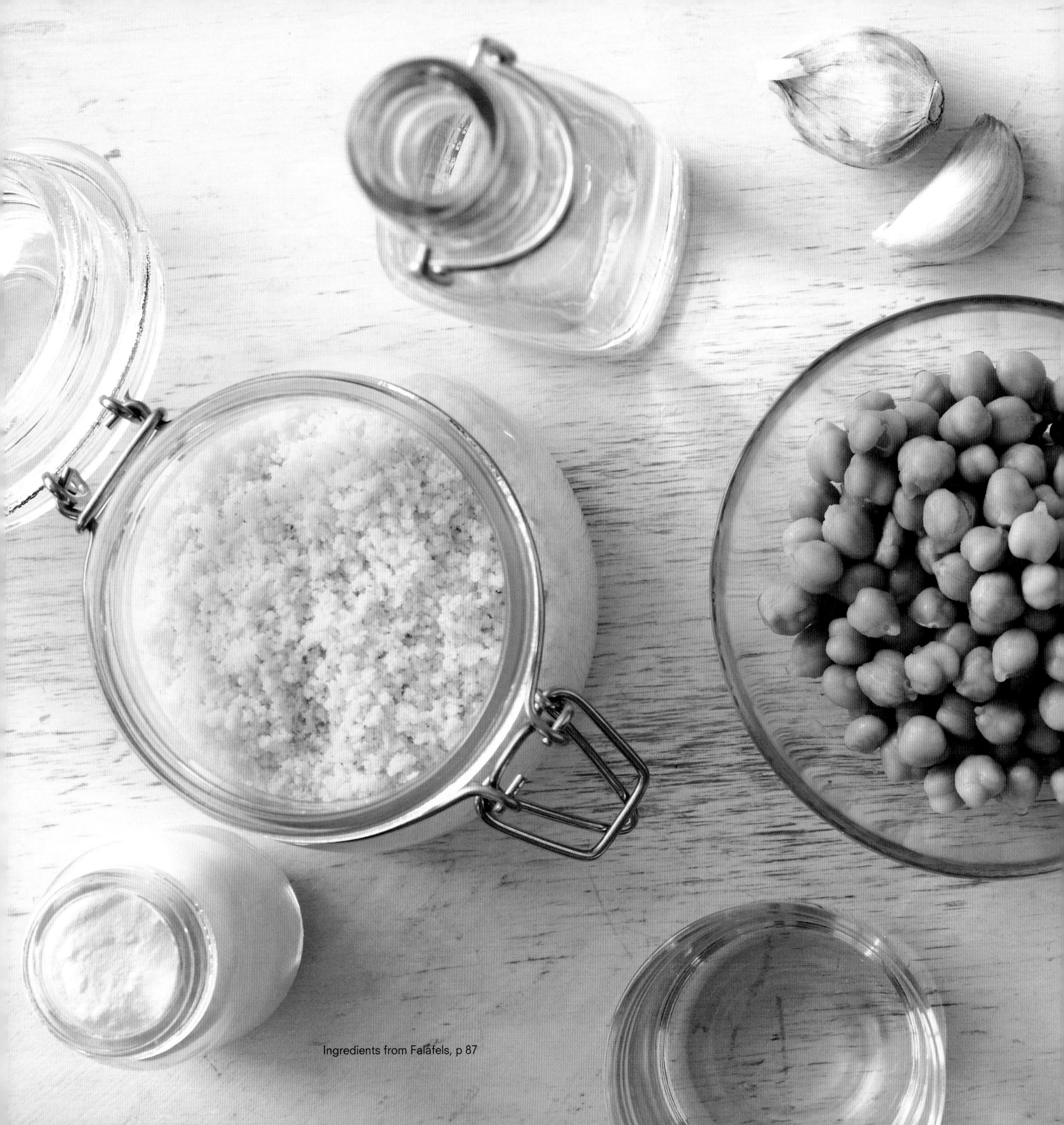

Ingredients from Falafels, p 87

vegetarian mains

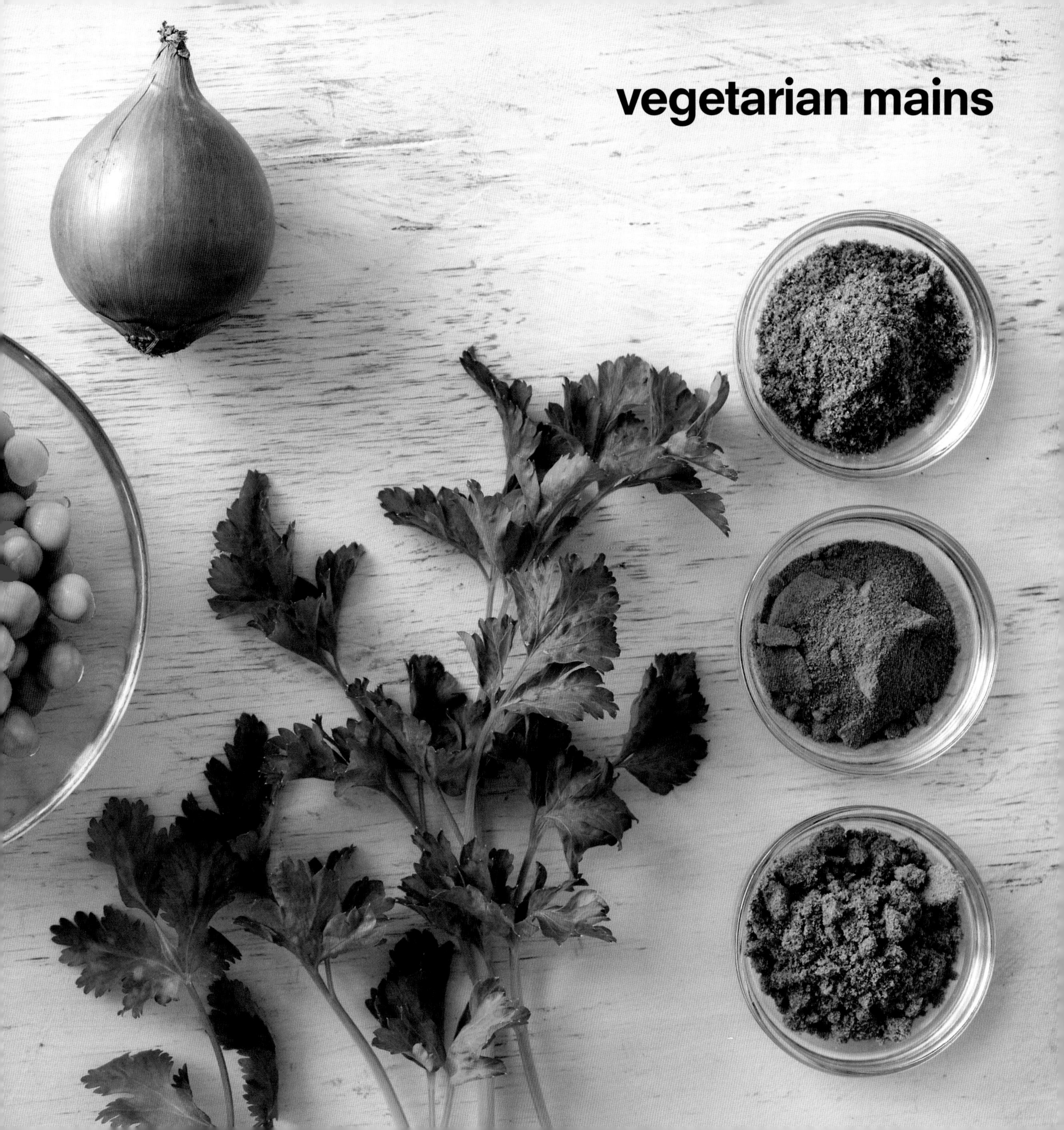

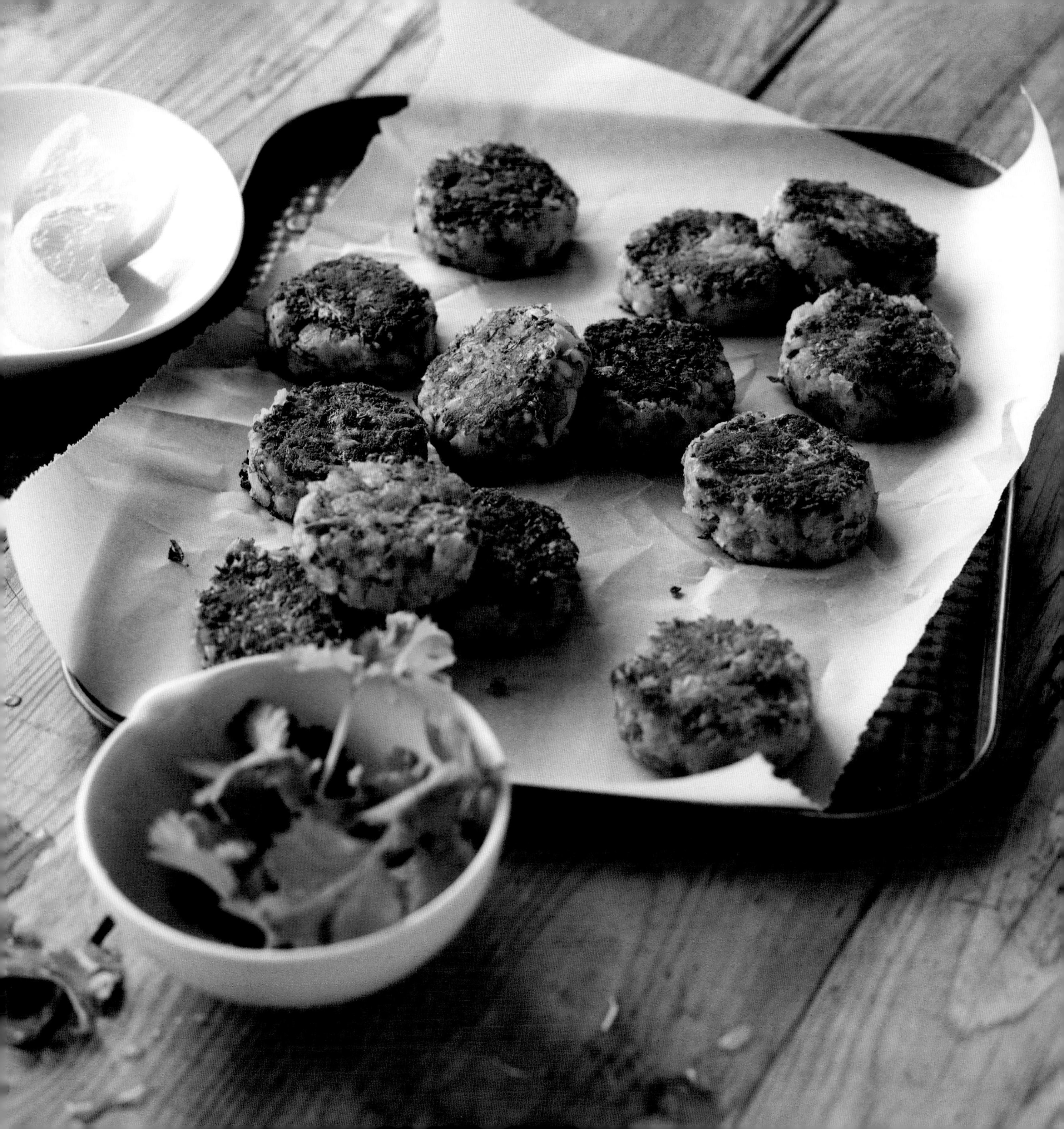

Falafels

Falafels are made from cooked, ground chickpeas shaped into balls or patties and deep-fried. The subtle flavour of the chickpeas is enhanced by aromatic Middle Eastern spices. These are lovely as a snack, but can be made into more of a meal by wrapping the falafels in a gluten-free, wheat-free, dairy-free, soy-free wrap with some salad.

MAKES 18

1 tablespoon olive oil
1 small onion, finely chopped
3 cloves garlic, crushed
1 tablespoon ground cumin
1 tablespoon ground coriander
¼ teaspoon ground turmeric
600 g tinned chickpeas, rinsed and drained
3 tablespoons chopped coriander
3 tablespoons chopped flat-leaf parsley
½ teaspoon baking powder
¾ cup (75 g) dried gluten-free, wheat-free, dairy-free, soy-free breadcrumbs
¾ teaspoon salt
¼ teaspoon freshly ground black pepper
vegetable oil, for shallow frying
lemon wedges and salad, to serve

Heat the olive oil in a small frying pan over medium heat. Add the onion, garlic, cumin, coriander and turmeric and cook, stirring, for 1 minute or until fragrant.

Place the chickpeas in a food processor and blend to a fine paste. Transfer to a large bowl. Add the spiced onion mixture, herbs, baking powder, breadcrumbs, salt and pepper and mix with your hands until well combined.

Shape the mixture into balls the size of large walnuts and flatten slightly. Place on a plate and refrigerate for 1 hour.

Pour the vegetable oil into a large, deep frying pan to a depth of 5 cm. Add the falafel in batches and cook, turning frequently, until golden brown all over. Remove with a slotted spoon and drain on paper towels. Serve hot with lemon wedges and salad.

Garlic and herb gnocchi with roast capsicum and tomato sauce

Making gnocchi from scratch can seem daunting, and it is often seen as a dish best ordered at a restaurant. However, it's worth being adventurous in the kitchen to make this one. It really isn't difficult and you'll be so pleased with the results. SERVES 4

1 kg desiree potatoes, cut into 2 cm cubes
salt and freshly ground black pepper
1 tablespoon chopped flat-leaf parsley, plus extra leaves to garnish
1½ tablespoons chopped basil
1½ tablespoons chopped chives
1 clove garlic, crushed
1 cup (180 g) potato flour
½ cup (50 g) maize cornflour, plus extra for dusting
1 egg yolk, lightly whisked*

ROAST CAPSICUM AND TOMATO SAUCE
3 red capsicums (peppers), seeded and cut into large pieces
4 roma (plum) tomatoes, cut in half
olive oil, for drizzling and pan-frying
1 clove garlic, crushed
1 onion, diced
1 cup (280 g) pureed tomato
1½ tablespoons chopped flat-leaf parsley
salt and freshly ground black pepper

Preheat the oven to 180°C

To make the sauce, place the capsicum and tomato halves on a large baking tray, drizzle with a little olive oil and bake for 20 minutes or until golden brown. If you want to remove the capsicum skins, put the capsicum in a plastic bag for a few minutes to steam, then peel off the skin. Cut the flesh into strips.

Heat 2 tablespoons olive oil in a medium frying pan over medium–low heat, add the garlic and onion and cook until golden brown. Increase the heat to medium–high. Add the roast capsicum and tomato and the pureed tomato and bring to the boil, then reduce the heat to medium–low and simmer for 15 minutes. Stir in the parsley and season with salt and pepper.

Meanwhile, cook the potato in a medium saucepan of boiling water until just tender. Drain and transfer to a large heatproof bowl. Mash with a potato masher until completely smooth, then season well with salt and pepper. Stir in the herbs and garlic.

Sift the flours into a small bowl and mix well with wooden spoon. Add 3 tablespoons flour and the egg yolk to the mashed potato and stir with a wooden spoon until combined. Stir in the remaining flour in two batches, then gently form into a soft dough. Place the dough on a benchtop dusted with cornflour and knead lightly.

Divide the dough into six equal portions. Roll one portion into a log about 30 cm long and 1 cm wide, then cut into 2 cm lengths. Repeat with the remaining dough.

Fill a large saucepan with water and bring to the boil over high heat. Add the gnocchi in small batches and cook for 3–4 minutes or until they rise to the surface. Remove with a slotted spoon, draining away any excess water, and place in a large bowl. Bring the water back to the boil between each batch.

Return the sauce to the heat and warm through if necessary. Divide the gnocchi among four bowls and spoon the sauce over the top. Garnish with parsley leaves and a grinding of pepper, then serve.

***For egg allergy**
Omit the egg yolk. Reduce the flours to ¾ cup (135 g) potato flour and ⅓ cup (50 g) maize cornflour. Sift 1 teaspoon xanthan gum with the flours and continue with the recipe.

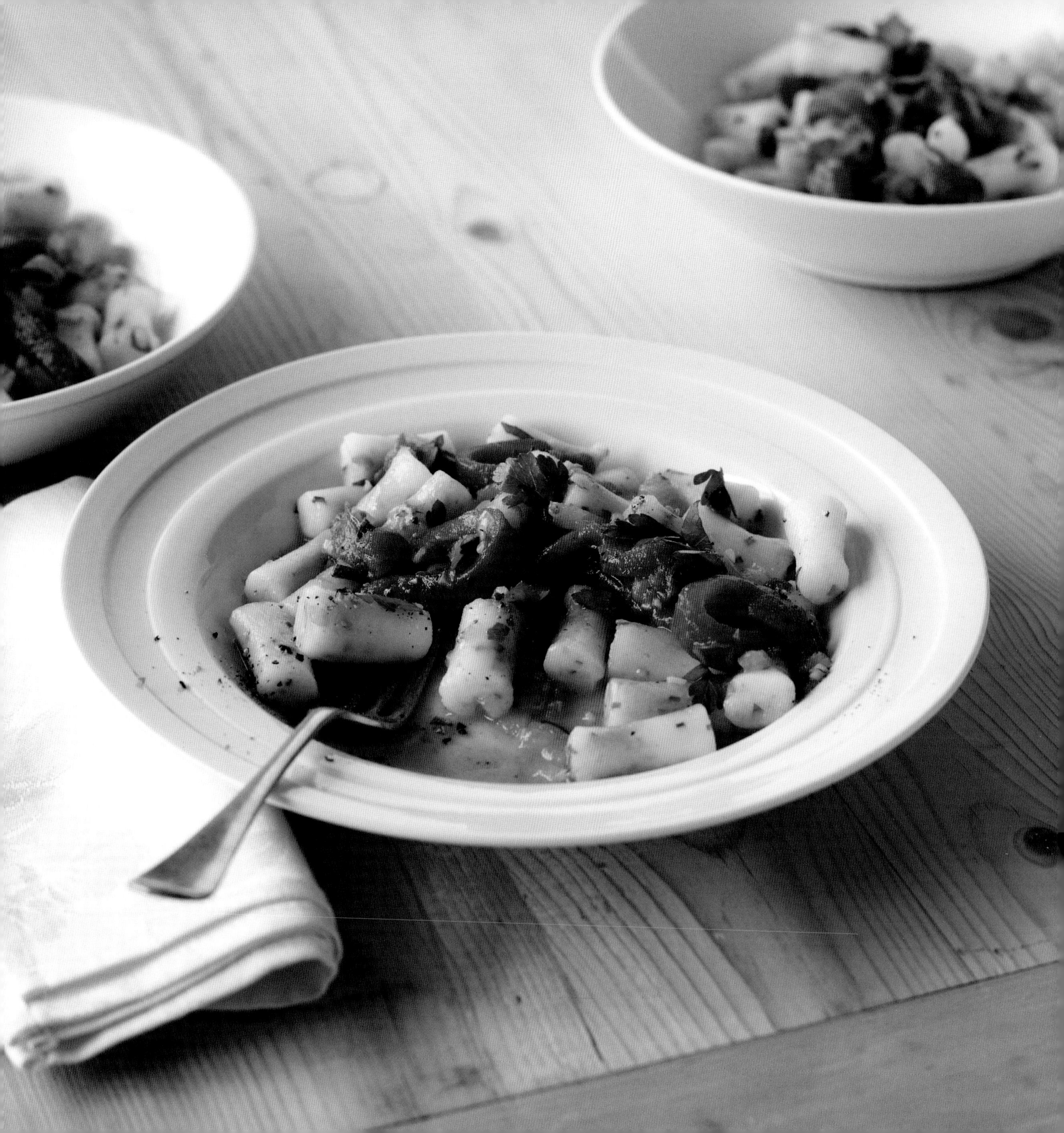

Chickpeas with ratatouille

Ratatouille is packed with flavour, and adding protein-rich chickpeas makes it a complete vegetarian meal. Enjoy it on its own or serve it with steamed brown rice or garlic and rosemary polenta (see page 64). SERVES 4

1 tablespoon olive oil
2 cloves garlic, crushed
1 onion, chopped
3 large zucchinis (courgettes), chopped
1 large red capsicum (pepper), seeded and chopped
2 medium eggplants (aubergines), chopped
1 × 400 g tin chickpeas, rinsed and drained
1 × 400 g tin chopped tomatoes
¼ teaspoon chilli powder
2 tablespoons chopped flat-leaf parsley
2 teaspoons chopped oregano
salt and freshly ground black pepper

Heat the olive oil in a large heavy-based saucepan over medium heat, add the garlic and onion and cook for 1–2 minutes or until softened.

Add the zucchini, capsicum and eggplant and cook, stirring, until the vegetables have softened. Stir in the chickpeas, chopped tomatoes and chilli. Reduce the heat to medium–low and cook, stirring occasionally, for 15 minutes or until the mixture has thickened.

Remove from the heat and stir in the parsley and oregano. Season with salt and pepper and serve.

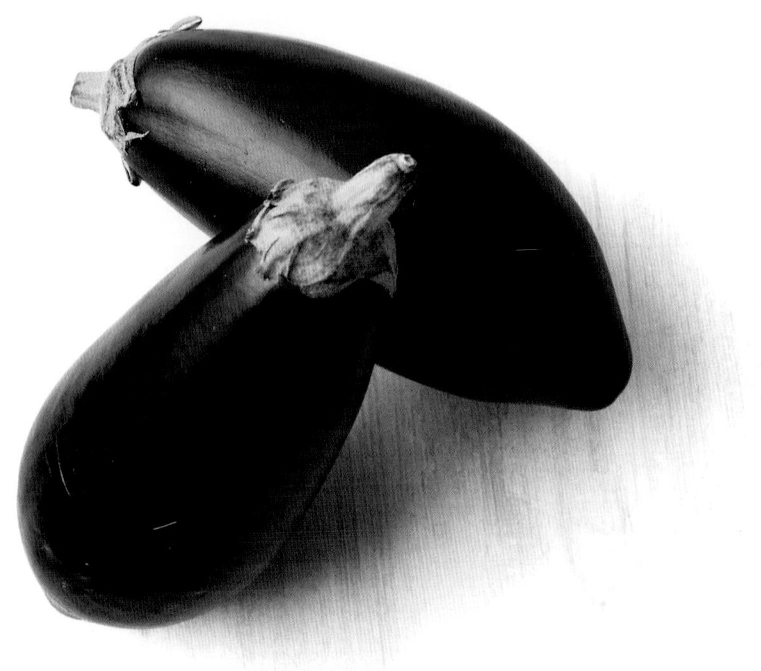

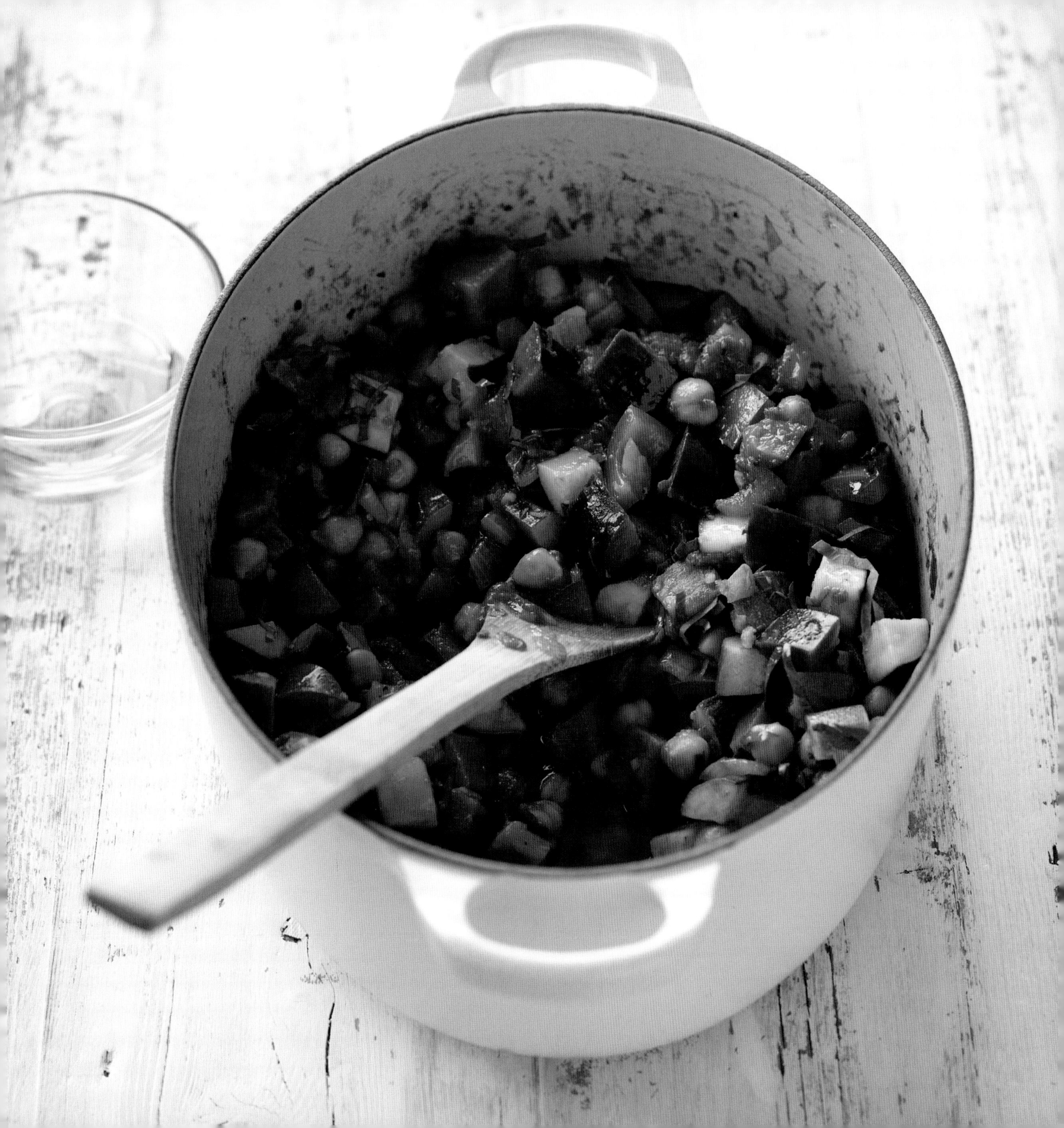

Spinach, pumpkin and sage polenta slice

I love the fact that polenta, when cooked firm as it is here, can be a base for so many flavour combinations. This time I'm enjoying the mix of sage, pumpkin and spinach, and I'm sure you will too. It's delicious served with garden salad with avocado (see page 22). SERVES 4

400 g pumpkin (squash), peeled and cut into 2 cm cubes
canola oil, for drizzling
3 cups (750 ml) gluten-free, wheat-free, dairy-free, soy-free vegetable stock
1 cup (170 g) instant polenta
2 cloves garlic, crushed
1½ tablespoons soy-free, dairy-free spread
2 tablespoons roughly chopped sage leaves
2 cups (60 g) baby spinach leaves
salt and freshly ground black pepper
green salad, to serve

Preheat the oven to 180°C.

Place the pumpkin pieces on a baking tray and drizzle with canola oil. Bake for 30–40 minutes or until cooked and golden, turning occasionally. Remove from the oven, then cover with foil and set aside.

Bring the stock to the boil in a medium saucepan. Add the polenta and garlic, then reduce the heat to medium–low and cook, stirring constantly, for 2–3 minutes. By this stage the mixture should be very thick. Remove the pan from the heat and stir through the dairy-free spread, sage and spinach until the spinach has wilted. Season to taste with salt and pepper.

Line a 20 cm square baking dish with baking paper and arrange the pumpkin pieces over the base. Pour the polenta mixture over the top and smooth the surface. Allow to cool slightly, then refrigerate for 2–3 hours or until firm.

Turn out the polenta onto a chopping board and cut into pieces. Enjoy it cold, or warm it under a medium grill on foil for 3–5 minutes. It's also delicious chargrilled. Serve with a green salad.

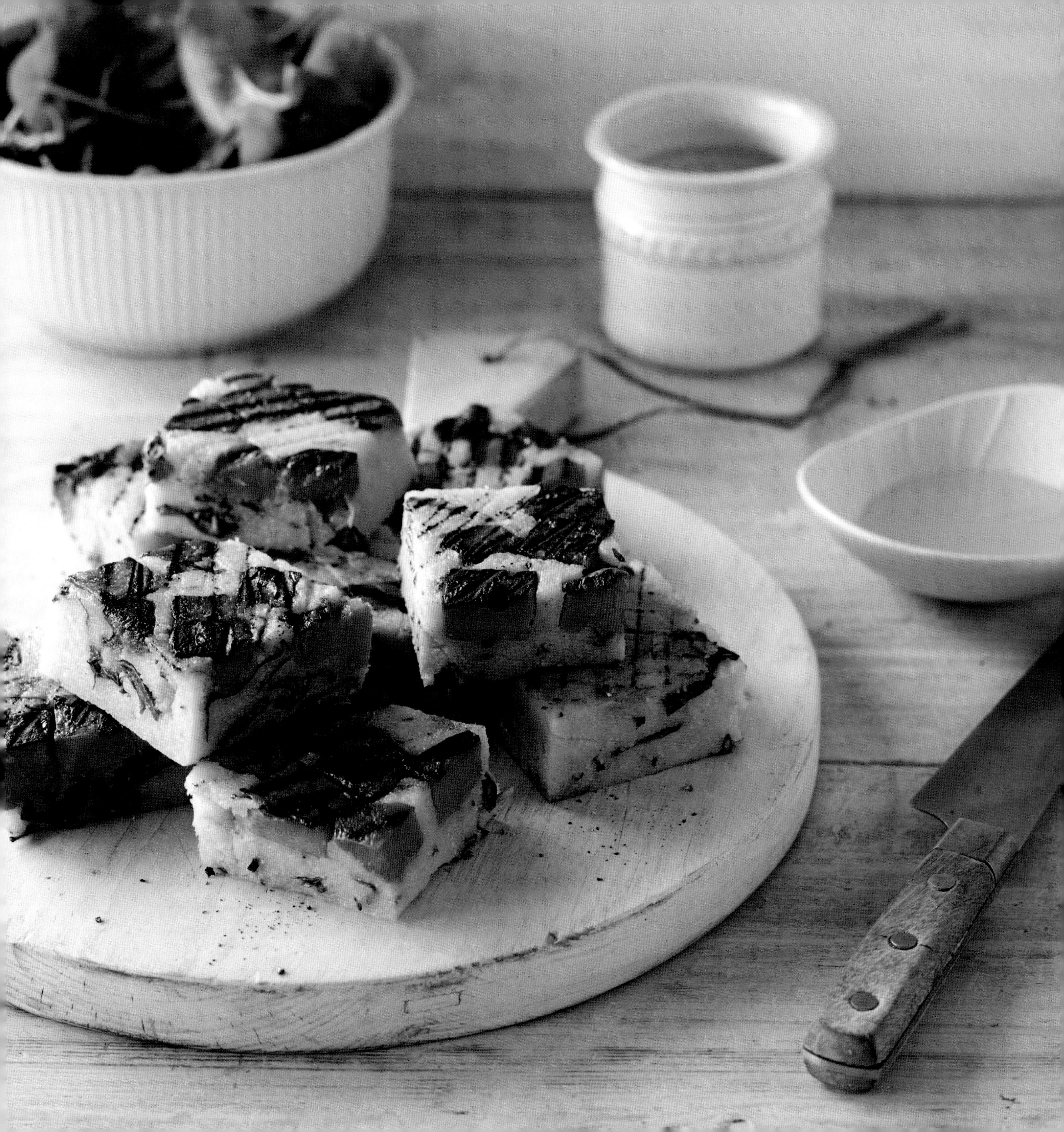

Lentil soup

Red lentils are suggested in the ingredients list, however brown lentils also work brilliantly in this wholesome soup. The vegetables add texture, flavour and vitamins, resulting in a cheering dish for a cold, wintery day. SERVES 4–6

1½ cups (300 g) red lentils
1 tablespoon olive oil
1 onion, chopped
3 cloves garlic, crushed
2 teaspoons thyme leaves
2 large potatoes, diced
3 large carrots, diced
1 large turnip, diced
3 sticks celery, chopped
1 small head cauliflower, chopped into small florets
2 bay leaves
2 litres gluten-free, wheat-free, dairy-free, soy-free vegetable stock
100 g chopped frozen spinach, thawed
2 tablespoons chopped flat-leaf parsley
salt and freshly ground black pepper

Soak the lentils in a large bowl of water for 2 hours. Drain.

Heat the olive oil in a large saucepan over medium–high heat, add the onion, garlic, thyme and drained lentils and cook for 2 minutes or until the onion has softened. Add the potato, carrot, turnip, celery, cauliflower, bay leaves and stock. Bring to the boil, then reduce the heat to medium–low and simmer, covered, for 1 hour or until the lentils are soft, stirring regularly.

Remove the pan from the heat and take out the bay leaves. Stir through the spinach and parsley and season to taste with salt and pepper.

Hearty vegetable soup >

There is a whole lot of goodness in each bowl of this tasty soup. You can add any other vegetables you happen to have – a great way to make sure they don't go to waste. SERVES 2

2 tablespoons olive oil
1 onion, diced
1 carrot, diced
1 stick celery, chopped
1 large potato, diced
3 cups (750 ml) gluten-free, wheat-free, dairy-free, soy-free vegetable stock
210 g tin chopped tomatoes
420 g tin white bean mix, rinsed and drained
50 g green beans, trimmed and cut into 1 cm lengths
1 large zucchini (courgette), diced
2 tablespoons finely chopped basil, plus extra shredded basil to garnish
¼–½ teaspoon dried chilli flakes (optional)
toasted gluten-free, wheat-free, dairy-free, soy-free bread, to serve (optional)

Heat the olive oil in a large saucepan over medium heat, add the onion and cook until softened. Add the carrot, celery and potato and cook for 2 minutes.

Increase the heat and add 1 cup (250 ml) stock. Bring to the boil, then reduce the heat to medium–low and simmer for 5 minutes or until the liquid has reduced by half. Add the chopped tomatoes, white beans, green beans, zucchini and remaining stock and cook for 2–3 minutes.

Remove the pan from the heat and stir in the basil and chilli flakes (if using). Garnish with extra basil, then serve immediately with toast, if liked.

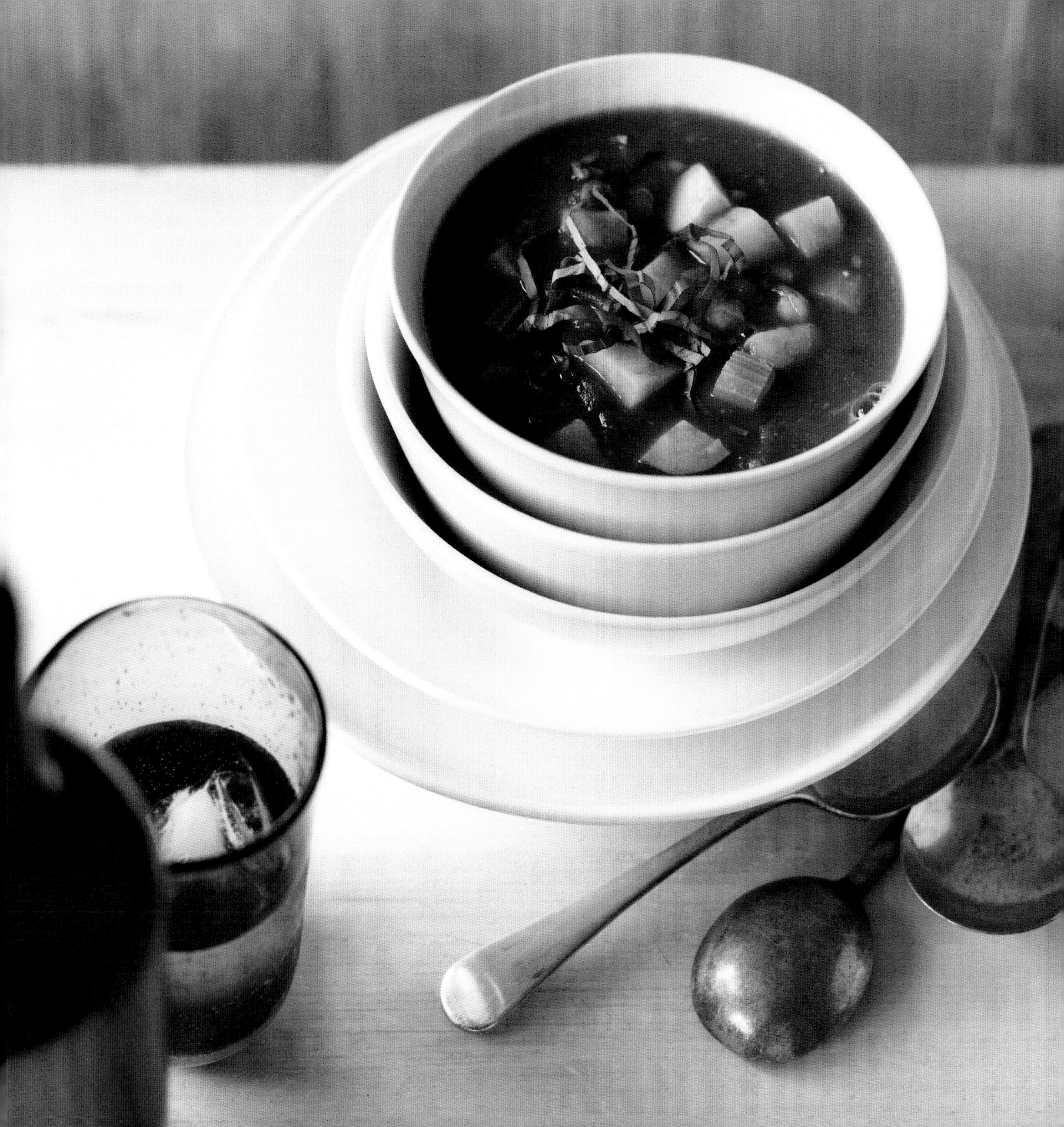

Thai pumpkin soup

This Asian twist on traditional pumpkin soup is divine. The creamy coconut complements the sweet, nutty pumpkin, and fresh coriander adds the final touch. If you are allergic to coconut, replace the coconut milk with rice milk.

SERVES 4

2 kg pumpkin (squash), peeled and cut into 2 cm pieces
1.5 litres strong gluten-free, wheat-free, dairy-free, soy-free vegetable stock
1 cup (250 ml) coconut milk, plus extra to serve (optional)
salt and freshly ground black pepper
⅓ cup chopped coriander

Preheat the oven to 180°C.

Place the pumpkin pieces in a large saucepan of boiling water and cook for 5–8 minutes or until softened. Drain and place in a large saucepan with the stock. Bring to the boil, then reduce the heat and simmer over medium–low heat for 15–20 minutes, stirring occasionally.

Remove from the heat and allow to cool slightly. Stir in the coconut milk, then puree with a hand-held blender until smooth. Warm through over medium heat if necessary, then season to taste with salt and pepper and stir through most of the coriander.

Ladle the soup into bowls, add a swirl of extra coconut milk (if using) and garnish with the remaining coriander.

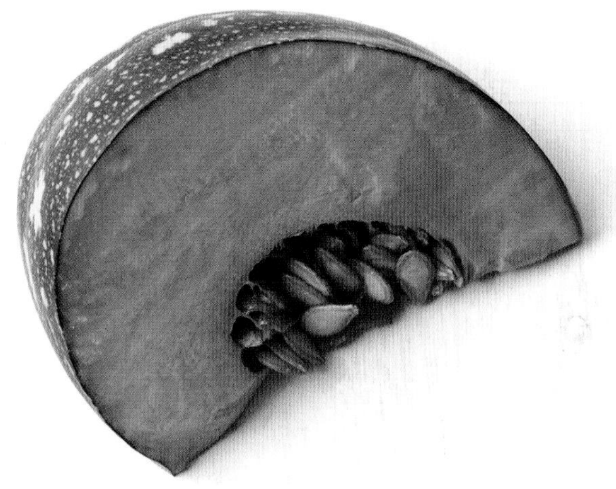

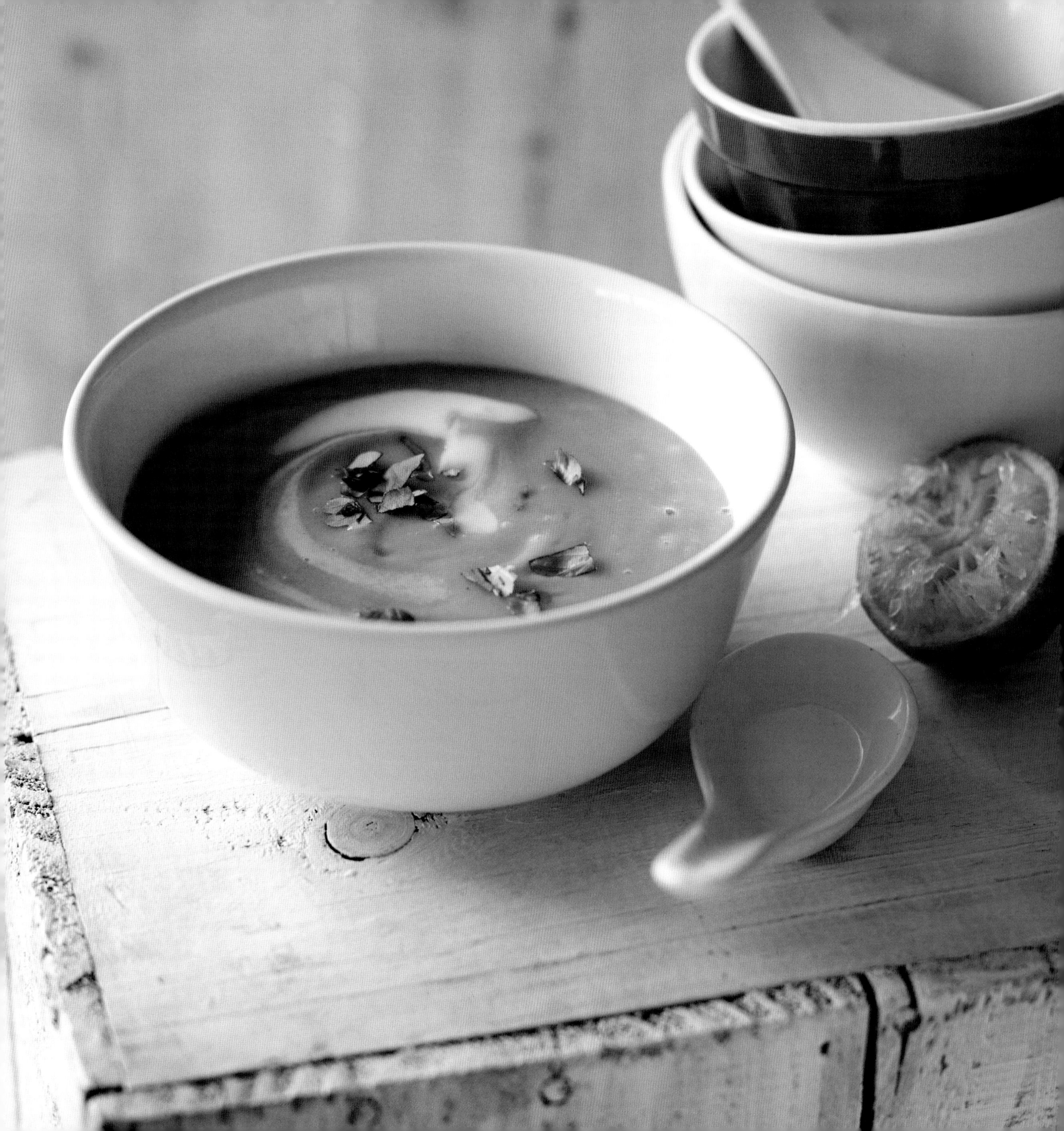

Curried spinach and capsicum kasha

Kasha is an Eastern European dish made from cooked buckwheat kernels. Buckwheat, despite the name, is another wheat-free, gluten-free grain and is highly versatile. Kasha is delicious served as a filling for baked potatoes, or with firm polenta. SERVES 4

2 tablespoons olive oil
2 cloves garlic, crushed
1 onion, finely sliced
1 teaspoon gluten-free, wheat-free curry powder
½ red capsicum (pepper), seeded and diced
1 cup (200 g) buckwheat kernels (or quinoa if unavailable)
3 cups (750 ml) gluten-free, wheat-free, dairy-free, soy-free vegetable stock
100 g chopped frozen spinach, thawed
3 tablespoons roughly chopped flat-leaf parsley
2–3 teaspoons gluten-free, wheat-free, dairy-free, soy-free fruit chutney
salt and freshly ground black pepper
⅓ cup chopped coriander
2 tablespoons grated lemon zest

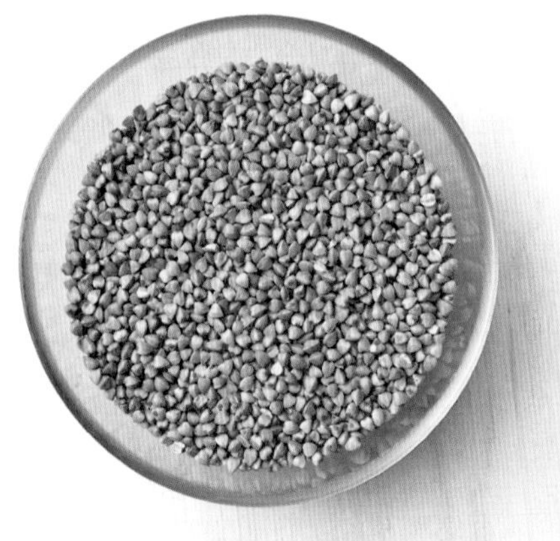

Heat the olive oil in a large non-stick frying pan over medium heat. Add the garlic, onion, curry powder and capsicum and cook until the onion has softened. Increase the heat to high. Add the buckwheat and stock and bring to the boil, then reduce the heat to low and simmer for 15–20 minutes, stirring occasionally, until most of the liquid has been absorbed and the buckwheat is tender.

Stir in the spinach, parsley and chutney and allow to warm through. Season to taste with salt and pepper, then scatter over the coriander and lemon zest and serve.

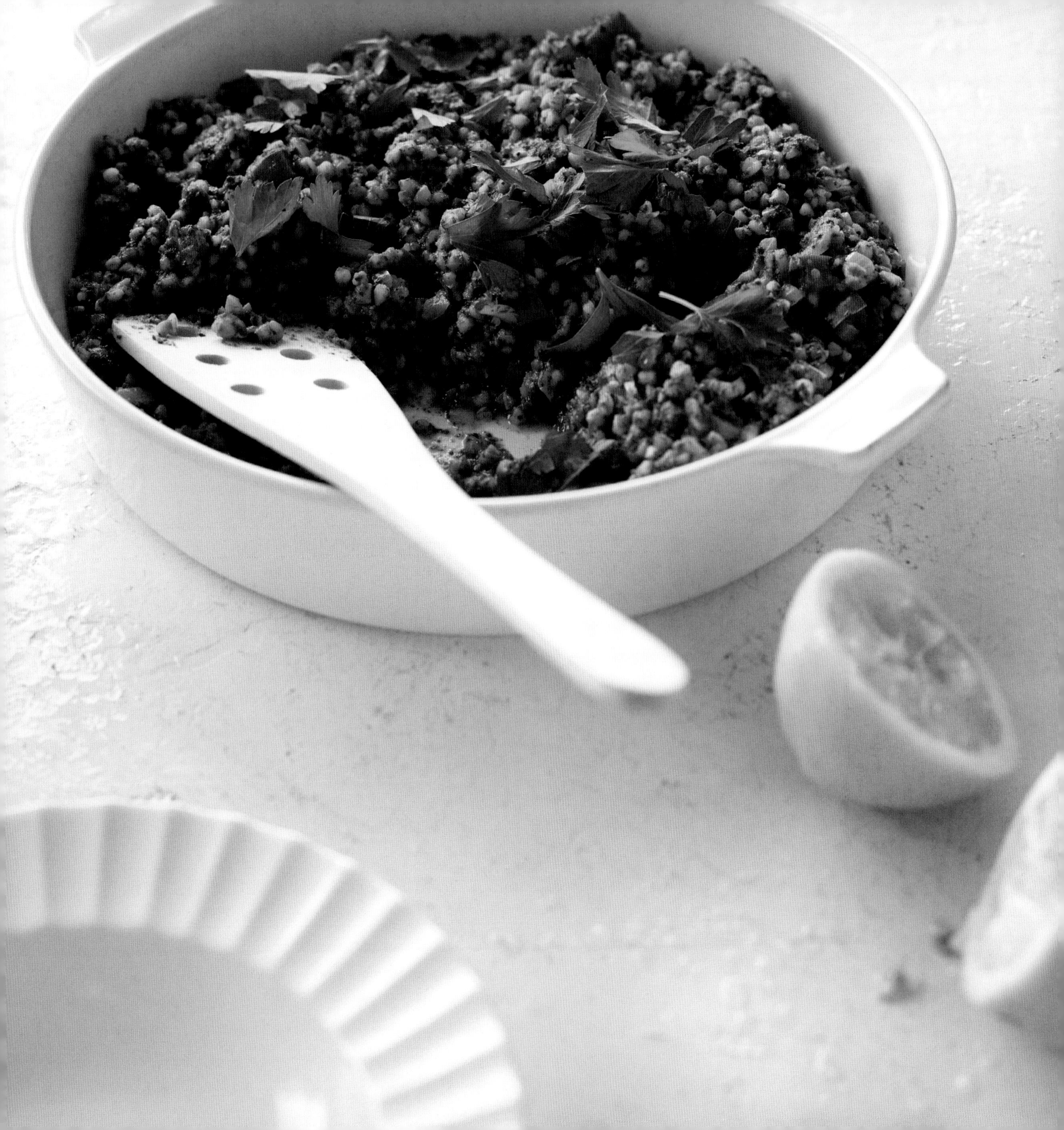

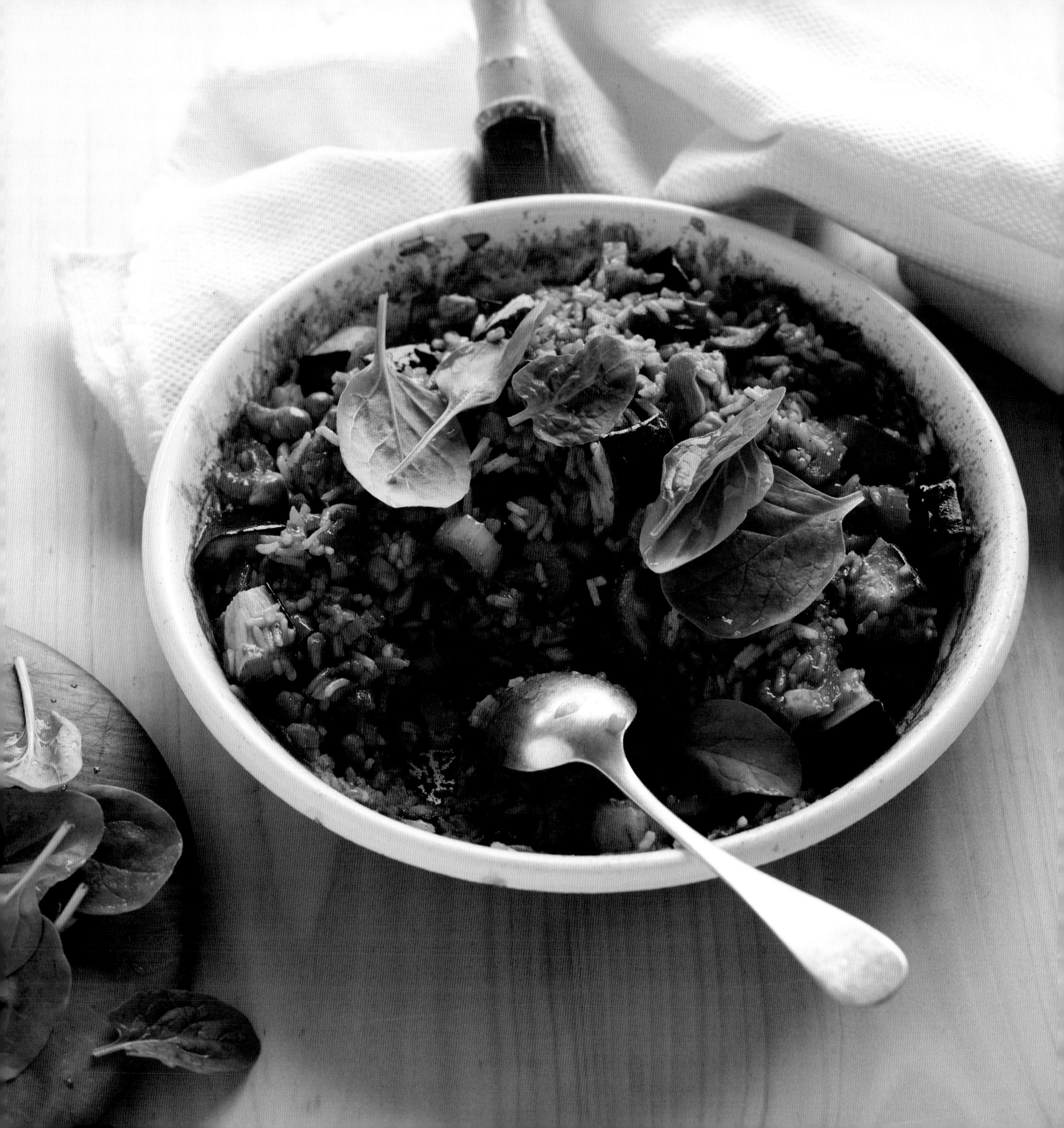

Roast eggplant pilaf with Middle Eastern spices

This vegetarian pilaf combines traditional Middle Eastern spices with roast eggplant. If you wish to adapt the recipe to include meat, add some sliced chicken, beef or lamb with the onion and saute until cooked. SERVES 4

450 g eggplant (aubergine), cut lengthways into 5 mm thick slices
olive oil, for drizzling and pan-frying
1 clove garlic, crushed
1 onion, chopped
3 teaspoons ground gluten-free, wheat-free, dairy-free, soy-free Middle Eastern spices
1 teaspoon ground turmeric
½–1 teaspoon chilli powder
3 cups (750 ml) gluten-free, wheat-free, dairy-free, soy-free vegetable stock (more if needed)
1 × 400 g tin chopped tomatoes
3 sticks celery, sliced
1½ cups (300 g) arborio rice
¾ cup (300 g) tinned chickpeas, drained
2 cups (60 g) baby spinach leaves

Preheat the oven to 180°C and line a baking tray with foil.

Place the eggplant slices on the tray and drizzle with a little olive oil. Bake for 15–20 minutes or until starting to turn golden brown. Remove and wrap in foil.

Heat 1 teaspoon olive oil in a large deep non-stick frying pan over medium–high heat. Add the garlic, onion, Middle Eastern spices, turmeric and chilli powder and cook until the onion has softened. Reduce the heat to medium–low. Add the stock, chopped tomatoes, celery and rice and simmer, covered, for 15–20 minutes or until the rice is tender (add extra stock if necessary). Turn off the heat.

Roughly chop the eggplant and add to the pan, along with the chickpeas and most of the spinach. Leave for a few minutes until the spinach has wilted, then serve, garnished with the remaining spinach leaves.

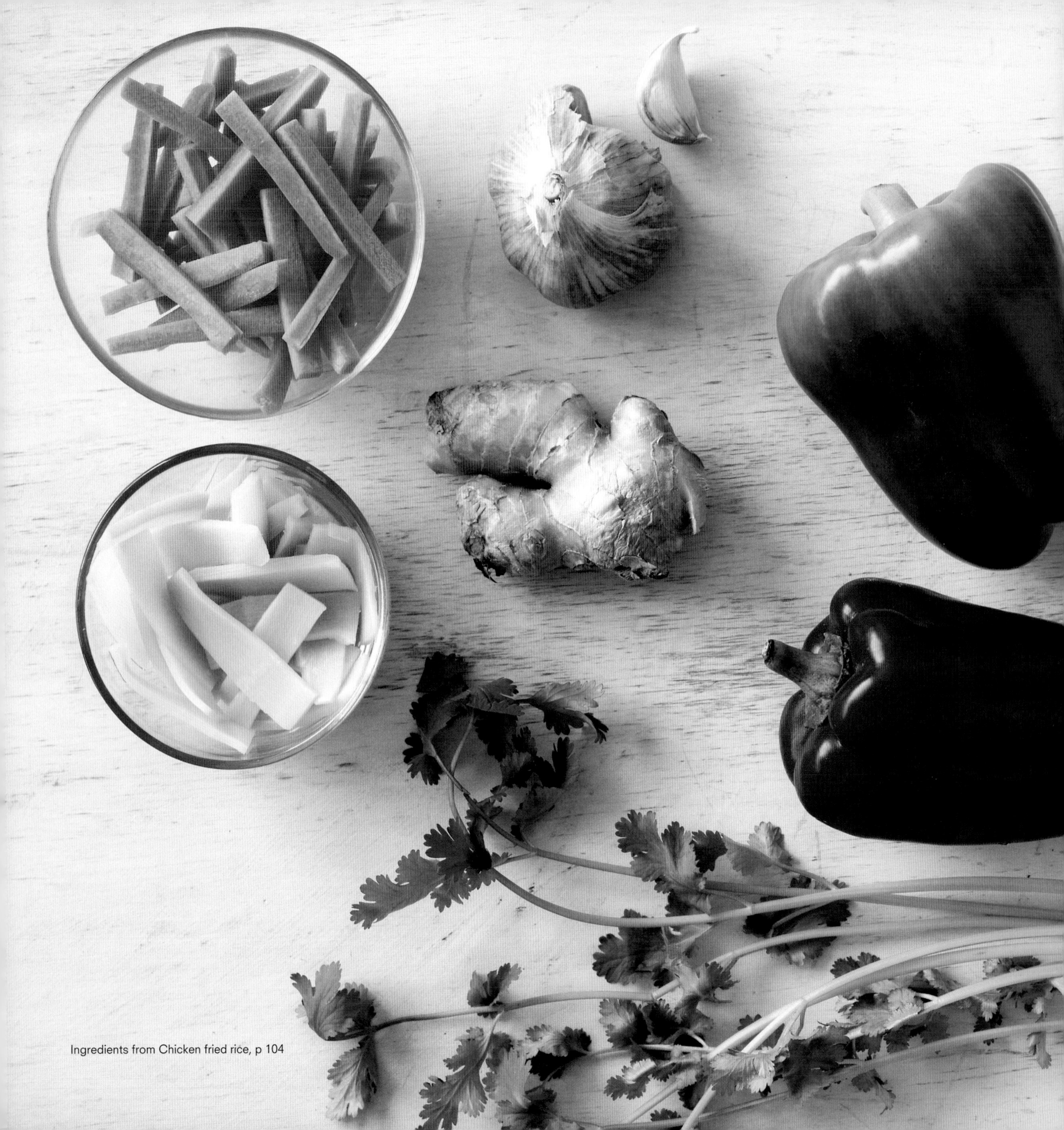

Ingredients from Chicken fried rice, p 104

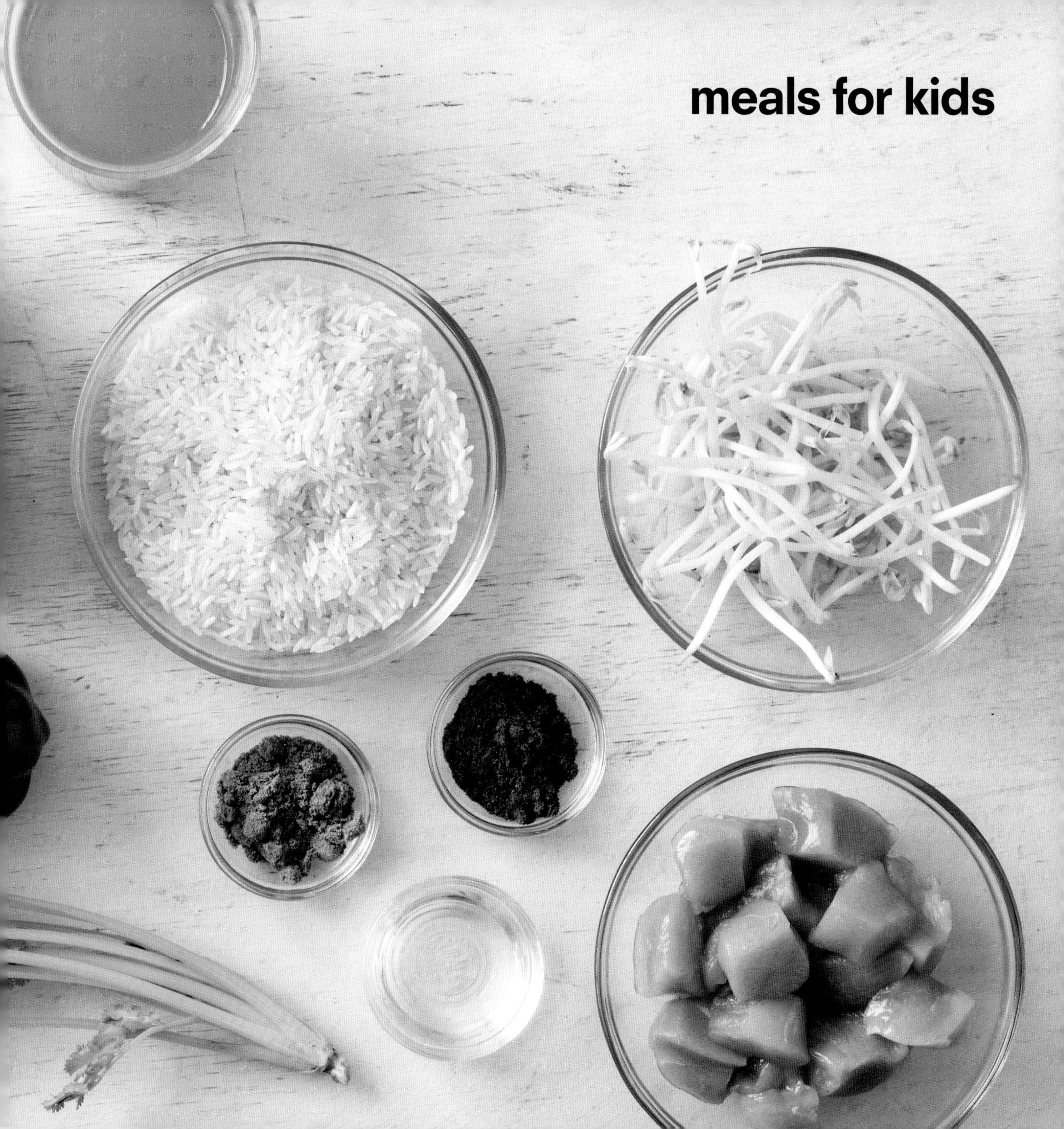
meals for kids

Chicken fried rice

The addition of chicken makes this traditional favourite a satisfying meal in a bowl. Cooking the rice in stock adds a delicious depth of flavour. SERVES 6

1.5 litres gluten-free, wheat-free, dairy-free, soy-free chicken stock
2 cups (400 g) long-grain rice
2 tablespoons canola oil
1½ teaspoons Chinese five-spice powder
½ teaspoon ground cumin
1½ tablespoons roughly chopped coriander
1 clove garlic, crushed
1 tablespoon grated ginger
500 g skinless chicken breast, sliced
1 carrot, cut into matchsticks
1 small green capsicum (pepper), thinly sliced into 2 cm lengths
1 small red capsicum (pepper), thinly sliced into 2 cm lengths
1 × 225 g tin bamboo shoots, drained
1 cup (80 g) bean sprouts
salt and freshly ground black pepper

Bring the stock to the boil in a large saucepan. Add the rice and cook for 10–12 minutes or until just tender. Drain.

Meanwhile, heat 1 tablespoon canola oil in a large wok or frying pan over medium heat, add the five-spice powder, cumin, coriander, garlic and ginger and cook until fragrant. Add the sliced chicken and toss for a few minutes until just browned. Add the carrot, capsicum, bamboo shoots and most of the bean sprouts and cook until the vegetables are tender.

Add the rice and toss until well combined. Finally, add the remaining canola oil, then taste and season with salt and pepper. Serve immediately, garnished with the remaining bean sprouts.

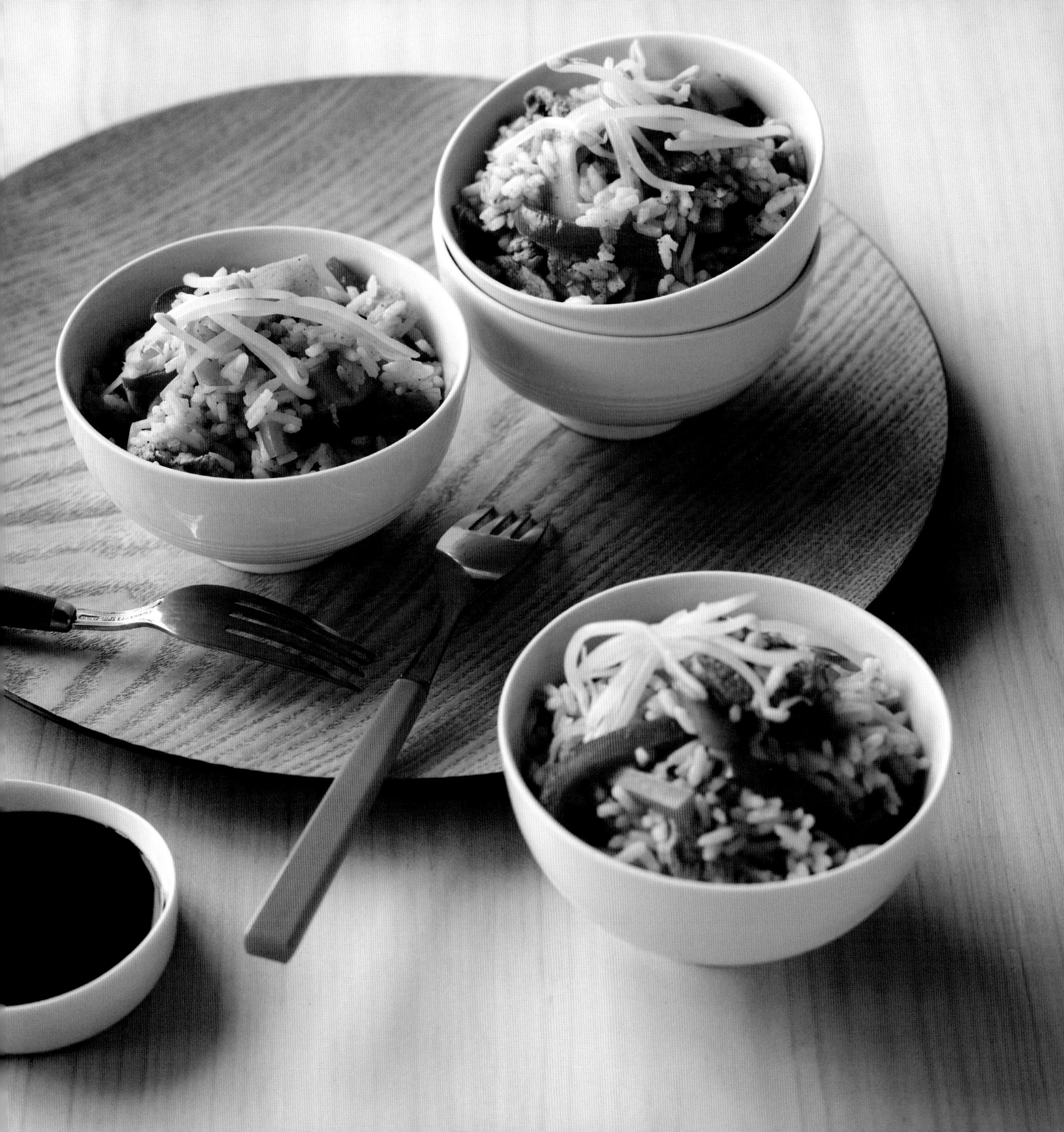

Porcupine meatballs

The rice sticks out of these meatballs, making them look like little porcupines. Perhaps we should call them echidna balls in Australia! Serve with allergy-free pasta or garlic and rosemary polenta (see page 64) and salad.

SERVES 4

½ cup (100 g) long-grain rice
2 cloves garlic, crushed
1 small onion, diced
1 tablespoon olive oil
750 g lean minced beef
½ cup (50 g) gluten-free, wheat-free, dairy-free, soy-free breadcrumbs
2 eggs, lightly beaten*
1 tablespoon finely chopped flat-leaf parsley
½ teaspoon cayenne pepper
salt and freshly ground black pepper
3 cups (750 ml) gluten-free, wheat-free, dairy-free tomato pasta sauce
500 g gluten-free, soy-free penne*
rocket leaves, to garnish (optional)

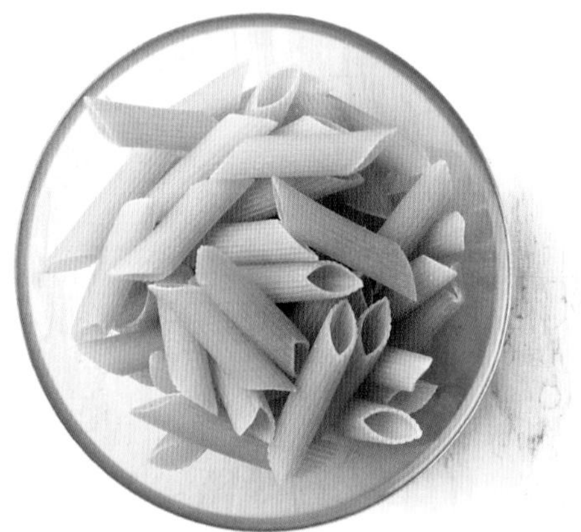

Cook the rice according to the packet instructions until tender. Drain and allow to cool.

Preheat the oven to 180°C.

In a large mixing bowl, combine the rice, garlic, onion, olive oil, mince, breadcrumbs, egg, parsley, cayenne pepper, salt and black pepper. Mix thoroughly, then shape into about 20 balls the size of golf balls.

Place in a large casserole dish and pour over the pasta sauce. Cover and bake for 40–50 minutes or until the meatballs are cooked through.

Shortly before the meatballs are ready, cook the pasta in a large saucepan of boiling water until just tender. Drain and serve with the meatballs and sauce, garnished with rocket leaves if liked.

***For egg allergy**

Place 2 teaspoons psyllium husks in a small bowl and pour over ½ cup (125 ml) boiling water, stirring constantly to ensure the psyllium does not clump together. Set aside for 4–5 minutes until it forms a gel, stirring occasionally. Use in place of the egg.

Make sure you use egg-free pasta.

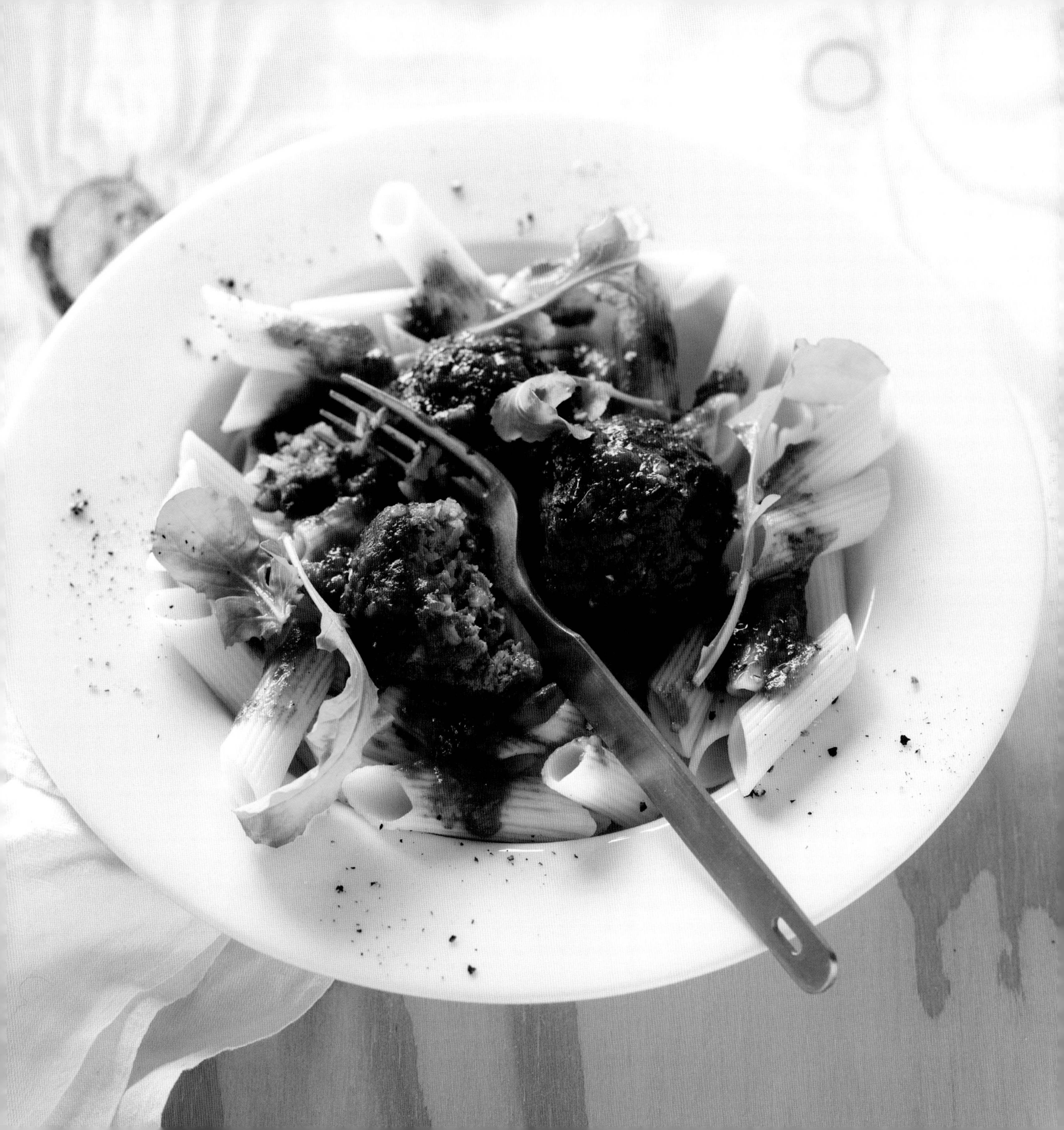

Meatloaf with tomato relish

Kids love meatloaf, and any leftovers work really well in the school lunchbox. For a hearty dinner, serve the meatloaf and relish with the sweet potato, prosciutto and green bean salad on page 26. SERVES 8

TOMATO RELISH

8 ripe tomatoes, peeled and sliced
1 large onion, thinly sliced
1½ tablespoons salt
2 teaspoons gluten-free, wheat-free, dairy-free, soy-free curry powder
1¼ teaspoons mustard powder
2 teaspoons maize cornflour
⅔ cup (170 ml) brown vinegar
¾ cup (165 g) firmly packed brown sugar
¼ teaspoon ground white pepper
¼ teaspoon ground ginger
¼ teaspoon grated nutmeg
pinch of chilli powder (optional)

MEATLOAF

400 g minced veal
400 g lean minced beef
⅔ cup (70 g) dried gluten-free, wheat-free, dairy-free, soy-free breadcrumbs
1 small onion, finely chopped
150 g lean bacon rashers, chopped
2 cloves garlic, crushed
2 small zucchinis (courgettes), grated
200 ml rice milk
¼ teaspoon grated nutmeg
¼ teaspoon cayenne pepper
1 egg*
salt and freshly ground black pepper

To make the relish, place the tomato, onion and salt in a medium saucepan filled with boiling water. Simmer over low heat for 15 minutes, then drain the water away, reserving the tomato mixture.

Mix the curry powder, mustard powder and cornflour in a small bowl. Add 2 tablespoons vinegar and mix to a smooth paste.

Add the remaining vinegar to the tomato mixture in the pan and bring to the boil over medium–high heat. Reduce the heat to medium–low and stir in the sugar and curry and mustard paste, then simmer for 30–40 minutes or until sauce is quite thick. Stir through the pepper, ginger, nutmeg and chilli (if using), then remove from the heat and set aside to cool. Spoon into an airtight jar and store in the fridge for up to 7 days.

Preheat the oven to 180°C. Grease a 23 cm × 13 cm × 7 cm loaf tin.

Combine all the meatloaf ingredients in a large bowl, then press into the loaf tin and bake for 50–60 minutes or until firm to the touch and cooked through. Remove from the oven and cover with foil, then leave to rest for 10–15 minutes

To serve, invert the meatloaf onto a board and cut into 2 cm thick slices. Serve hot or cold with the tomato relish and salad (if liked).

***For egg allergy**
Place 2 teaspoons psyllium husks in a small bowl and pour over ½ cup (125 ml) boiling water, stirring constantly to ensure the psyllium does not clump together. Set aside for 4–5 minutes until it forms a gel, stirring occasionally. Use in place of the egg.

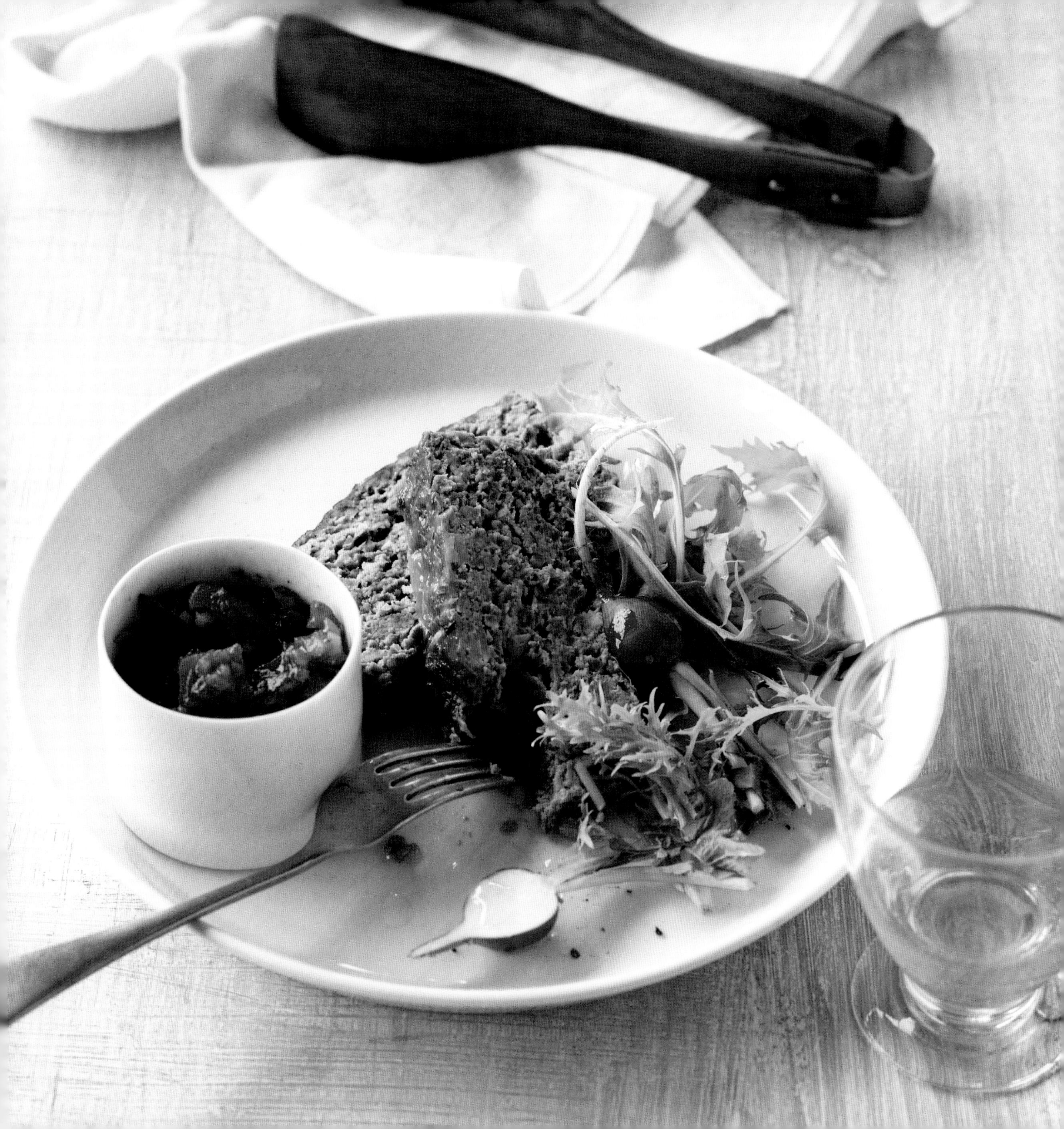

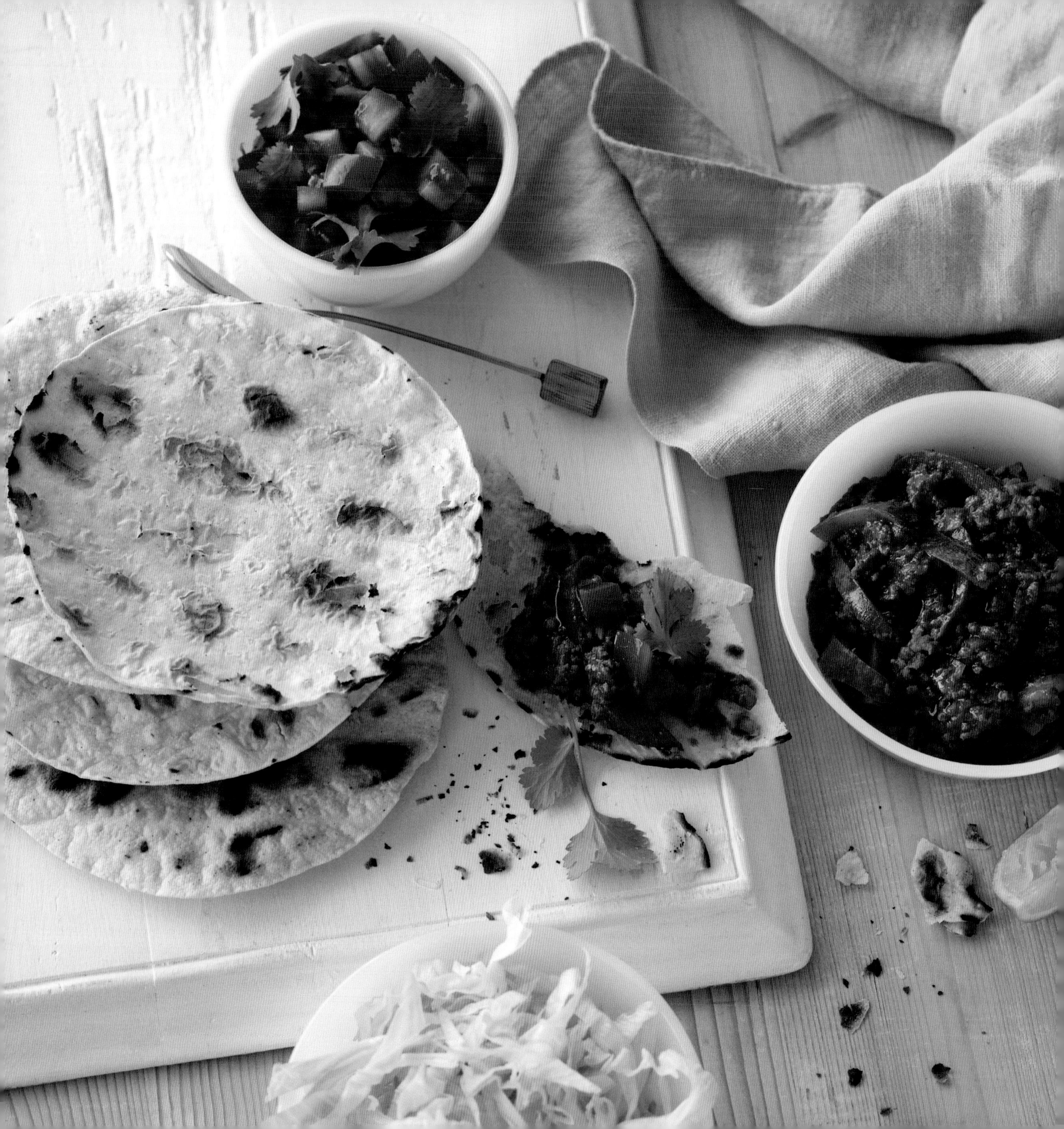

Beef burritos

Burritos are a popular Mexican dish, where meat is wrapped in a tortilla. In my recipe, I use gluten-free, wheat-free, dairy-free, soy-free wraps instead but the concept is the same. People who are not allergic to dairy products may wish to top the filling with grated cheese.

SERVES 4

8 maize gluten-free, wheat-free, dairy-free, soy-free tortillas
1 × 420 g tin red kidney beans, rinsed and drained
1½ teaspoons sweet paprika
1½ teaspoons ground cumin
1 teaspoon cayenne pepper
1–2 teaspoons chilli powder (optional)
¾ cup (250 g) tinned crushed tomatoes
2 teaspoons canola oil
1 small onion, diced
2 cloves garlic, crushed
700 g lean minced beef
1 zucchini (courgette), cut into thin 3 cm long strips
½ red capsicum (pepper), cut into thin strips
salt and freshly ground black pepper
½ iceberg lettuce, washed and shredded
2 ripe tomatoes, chopped
3 tablespoons coriander leaves
lime wedges to serve, optional

Preheat the oven to 180°C.

Wrap the tortillas in foil and heat in the oven for about 20 minutes. Alternatively, put them on a clean tea towel, sprinkle with a little water and heat in microwave for 1 minute 20 seconds on high just before serving.

Place the kidney beans, dried spices and crushed tomatoes in a food processor and process for 2 minutes or until nicely blended.

Heat the canola oil in a large frying pan over medium heat, add the onion, garlic and minced beef and cook until the meat is just browned. Pour the kidney bean puree over the top and stir in the zucchini and capsicum. Reduce the heat to medium–low and simmer for 7–10 minutes. Season to taste with salt and pepper.

Divide the shredded lettuce among the warmed tortillas. Top with spoonfuls of the beef mixture and sprinkle with chopped tomato and coriander leaves. Fold to encase the filling and serve with lime wedges, if liked.

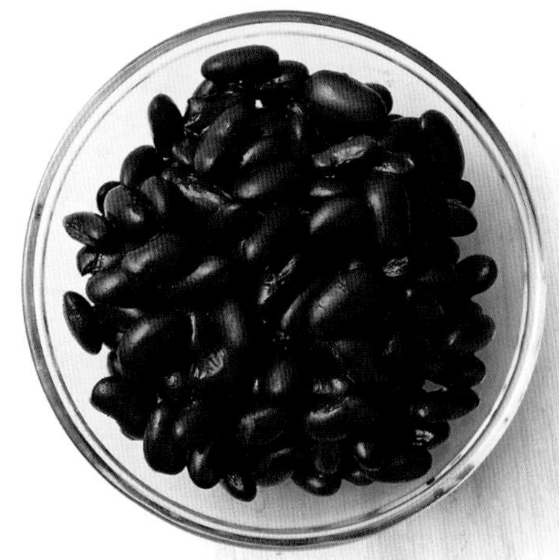

Curried sausage casserole

Sausages are often a favourite food for kids. Here, I've combined them with vegetables and a subtle curry sauce for a delicious, satisfying meal. SERVES 4–6

500 g plain gluten-free, wheat-free, dairy-free, soy-free pork sausages
2 teaspoons canola oil
1 small onion, diced
1 tablespoon gluten-free, wheat-free, dairy-free, soy-free curry powder
3 large potatoes, cut into 1 cm cubes
1 sweet potato (or 2 carrots), cut into 1 cm cubes
2 sticks celery, chopped
1 litre gluten-free, wheat-free, dairy-free, soy-free chicken stock
3 tablespoons gluten-free, wheat-free, dairy-free, soy-free gravy powder
steamed rice, to serve

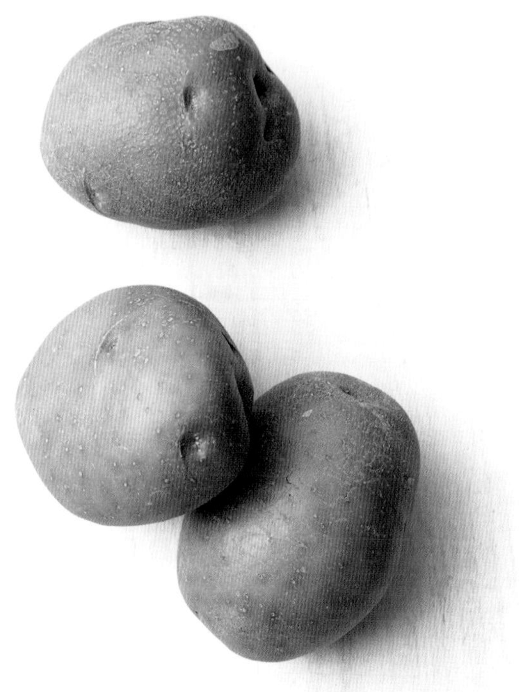

Cook the sausages in a non-stick frying pan over medium heat for 3–5 minutes, turning to ensure they are browned on all sides. Remove and cut into 1 cm thick slices.

Heat the canola oil in a large heavy-based saucepan over medium heat. Add the onion and curry powder and cook until the onion has softened. Add the sausage slices, potato, sweet potato and celery. Increase the heat to medium–high and add the stock and gravy powder. Bring to the boil, then reduce the heat to medium–low and simmer for 40 minutes, stirring occasionally, until the sauce has reduced and thickened. Serve with rice.

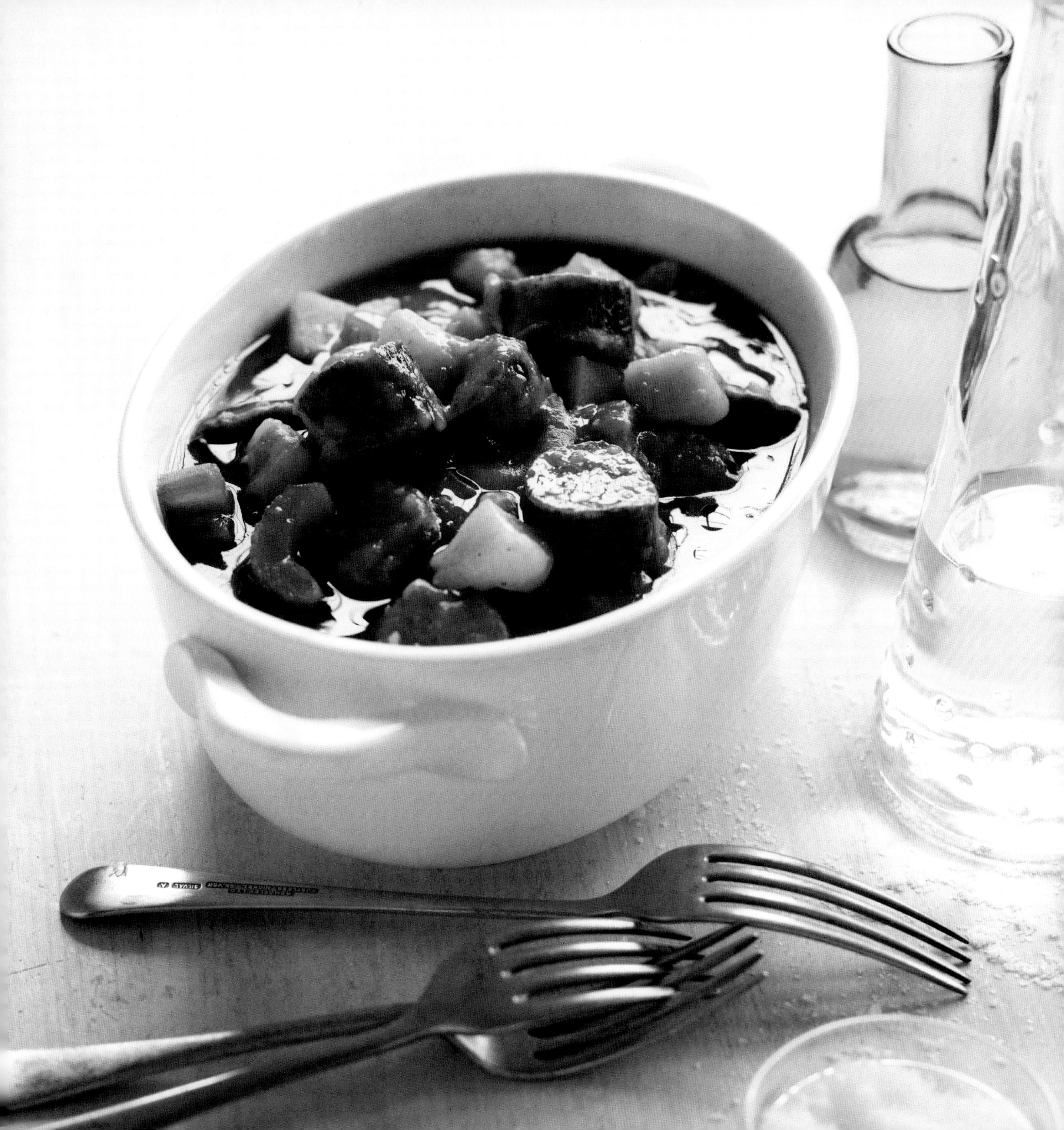

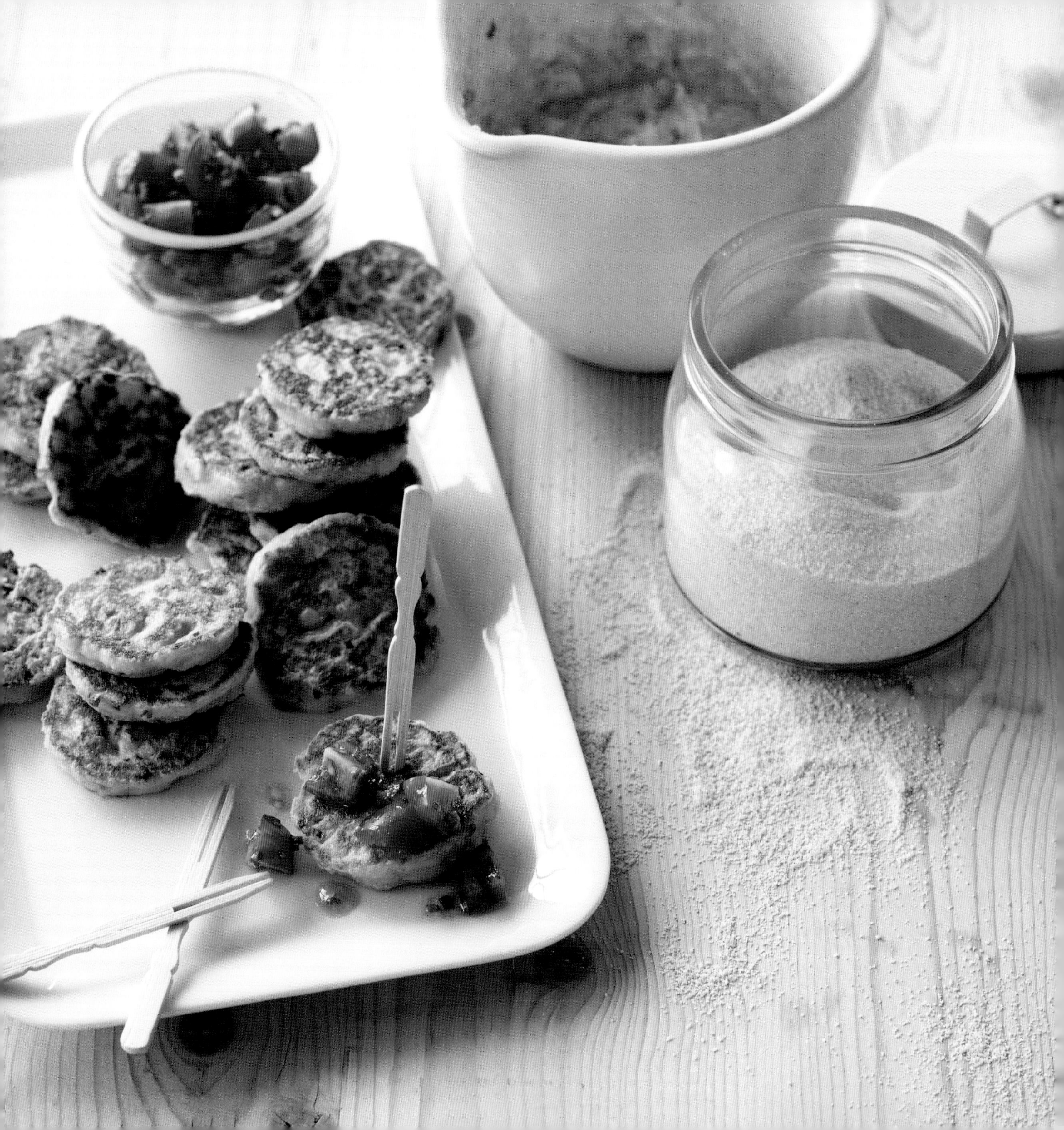

Corn fritters with fresh tomato salsa

Corn fritters are dangerously moreish and make the perfect savoury snack. The tomato salsa is a delicious, fresh accompaniment.

MAKES 16

⅓ cup (40 g) fine rice flour
3 tablespoons potato flour
3 tablespoons fine polenta
¼ teaspoon bicarbonate of soda
¼ teaspoon xanthan gum
⅔ cup (150 g) gluten-free, wheat-free creamed corn
1 tablespoon soy-free, dairy-free spread, melted
1 egg, lightly beaten*
1 tablespoon chopped flat-leaf parsley or chives
salt and freshly ground black pepper
cooking spray

FRESH TOMATO SALSA
250 g grape or cherry tomatoes, roughly chopped
½ cup finely chopped coriander
extra virgin olive oil, for drizzling
salt and freshly ground black pepper

Sift the flours, polenta, bicarbonate of soda and xanthan gum into a large bowl. Stir in the creamed corn, spread, egg and chopped herbs. Season with salt and pepper and set aside for 10 minutes.

To make the tomato salsa, place the tomato and coriander in a small bowl. Add a drizzle of olive oil and season to taste with salt and pepper, then toss gently to combine.

Heat a large heavy-based frying pan over medium heat and spray with cooking spray. Working in batches, spoon in 1 tablespoon batter for each fritter and cook for 2–3 minutes each side or until light brown and just cooked through. Transfer to plate and cover to keep warm. Repeat with the remaining batter, then serve the fritters warm with the tomato salsa.

***For egg allergy**
Place 1 teaspoon psyllium husks in a small bowl and pour over 3 tablespoons boiling water, stirring constantly to ensure the psyllium does not clump together. Set aside for 4–5 minutes until it forms a gel, stirring occasionally. Use in place of the egg.

Herbed wedges

Although this recipe has landed in the kids' chapter, grown-ups love these wedges too! They can be enjoyed on their own as a snack, or as a side to a steak or chicken meal. SERVES 4

2 tablespoons maize cornflour
1 teaspoon gluten-free, wheat-free, dairy-free, soy-free chicken stock powder
1 teaspoon finely chopped rosemary
½ teaspoon finely chopped oregano
½ teaspoon garlic powder
½ teaspoon salt
8 new potatoes, washed, skin left on
2 tablespoons olive oil

Preheat the oven to 200°C. Line a baking tray with baking paper.

In a plastic bag, combine the cornflour, stock powder, rosemary, oregano, garlic powder and salt.

Cut each potato into eight wedges. Add to the bag and toss in the seasoned flour, then shake off any excess. The potatoes should only be lightly coated.

Place the wedges in a single layer on the baking tray and brush with olive oil. Bake for 15 minutes, then reduce the temperature to 180°C and bake for a further 20 minutes or until crisp and golden brown, turning halfway through. Serve hot.

Lemon pepper chicken legs >

Delicately flavoured, fun and easy to eat, these are a great kids' meal. Serve with mash or potato wedges and salad or steamed vegetables. SERVES 4

½ teaspoon maize cornflour
⅓ cup (80 ml) lemon juice
2 cloves garlic, crushed
1 tablespoon grated lemon zest
1 teaspoon mustard powder
½–1 teaspoon finely ground black pepper
2 tablespoons canola oil
2 teaspoons finely chopped flat-leaf parsley
8 medium chicken drumsticks
lemon halves, to serve

In a small saucepan, blend the cornflour with the lemon juice to make a smooth paste. Add the garlic, lemon zest, mustard powder, pepper and canola oil and stir over medium–low heat until the sauce thickens. Allow to cool to room temperature, and then stir in the parsley.

Place the chicken drumsticks in a large baking dish, pour over the marinade and brush to make sure each drumstick is well coated. Cover and place in the fridge for a few hours.

Preheat a grill plate, chargrill pan or barbecue to medium–high. Cook the drumsticks, turning occasionally, for 10–12 minutes or until the juices run clear when the thickest part is pierced with a skewer. Alternatively, bake the drumsticks in a preheated 180°C oven for 20–25 minutes. Char the lemon halves on the grill, if liked, and serve with the drumsticks.

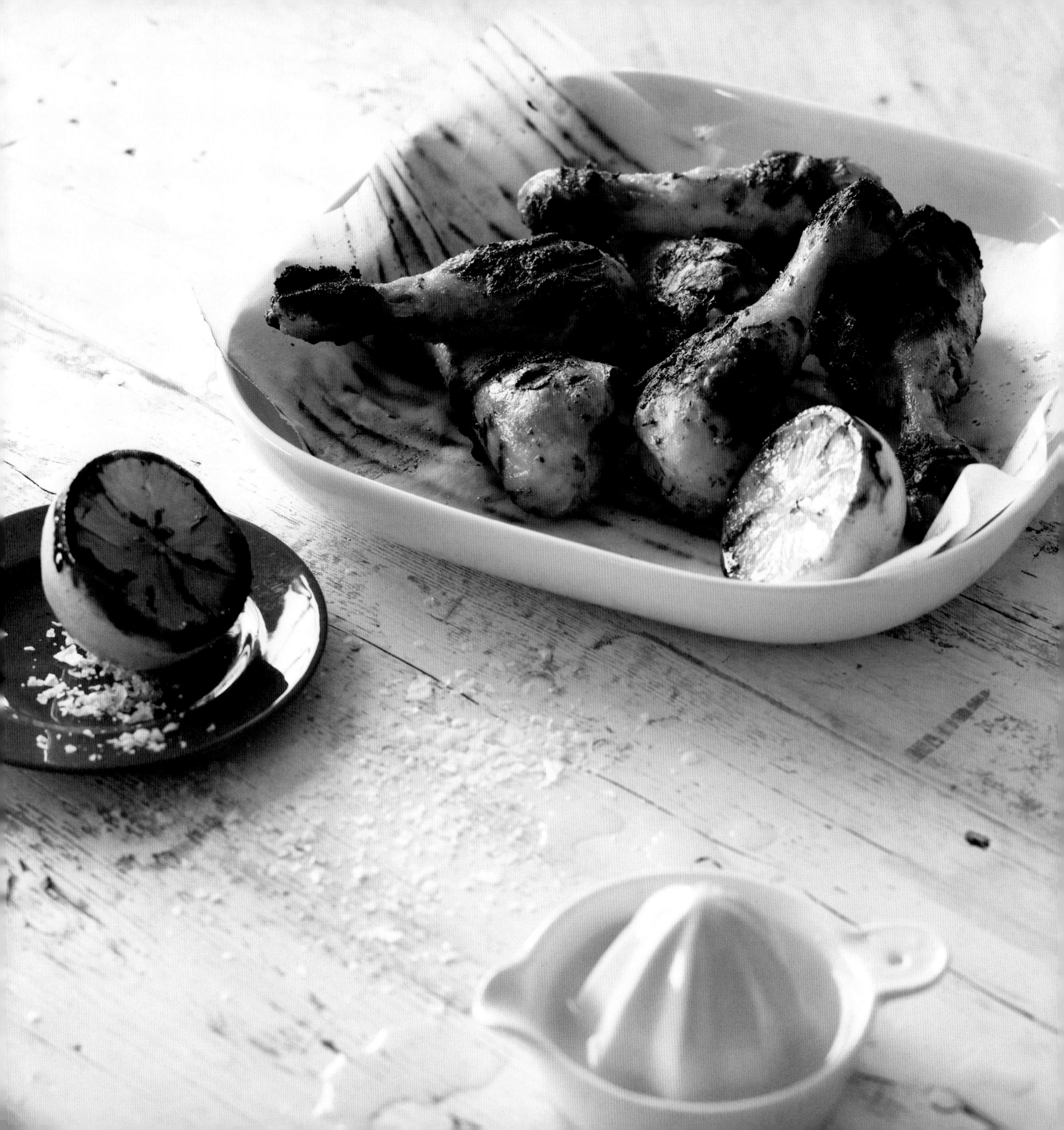

Pork spare ribs

This popular dish is difficult to order free of allergens in restaurants, so making it at home is probably your best bet. Although this recipe has sherry in it, the alcohol evaporates during the cooking process so it is safe to offer to children.

SERVES 4

2 tablespoons canola oil
3 cloves garlic, crushed
2–3 teaspoons finely chopped ginger
2–3 teaspoons maize cornflour
¾ cup (185 ml) gluten-free, wheat-free, dairy-free, soy-free chicken stock
3 tablespoons sherry
2½ teaspoons gluten-free, wheat-free soy sauce*
3 star anise
1 tablespoon brown sugar
2 kg pork spare ribs
steamed rice, to serve
sliced red chilli, to serve (optional)

Heat the canola oil in a medium saucepan over medium–low heat. Add the garlic and ginger and cook for 1–2 minutes or until fragrant.

Place the cornflour in a medium bowl and blend with a little stock to make a paste. Stir in the sherry, soy sauce, star anise, brown sugar and remaining stock. Add to the garlic and ginger in the pan and bring almost to the boil, stirring constantly, until the sauce is thick enough to coat the back of a spoon. Remove from the heat and leave to cool to room temperature. Remove the star anise.

Line a baking dish with baking paper. Add the spare ribs in a single layer and brush with the cooled sauce, making sure they are well coated on both sides. Cover and refrigerate for 2–3 hours.

Preheat the oven to 180°C.

Bake the ribs for 20–25 minutes or until cooked through. Serve with steamed rice and sliced chilli, if liked.

***For soy allergy**
In a small bowl, combine 2 teaspoons molasses and ½ teaspoon apple cider vinegar. Use in place of the soy sauce.

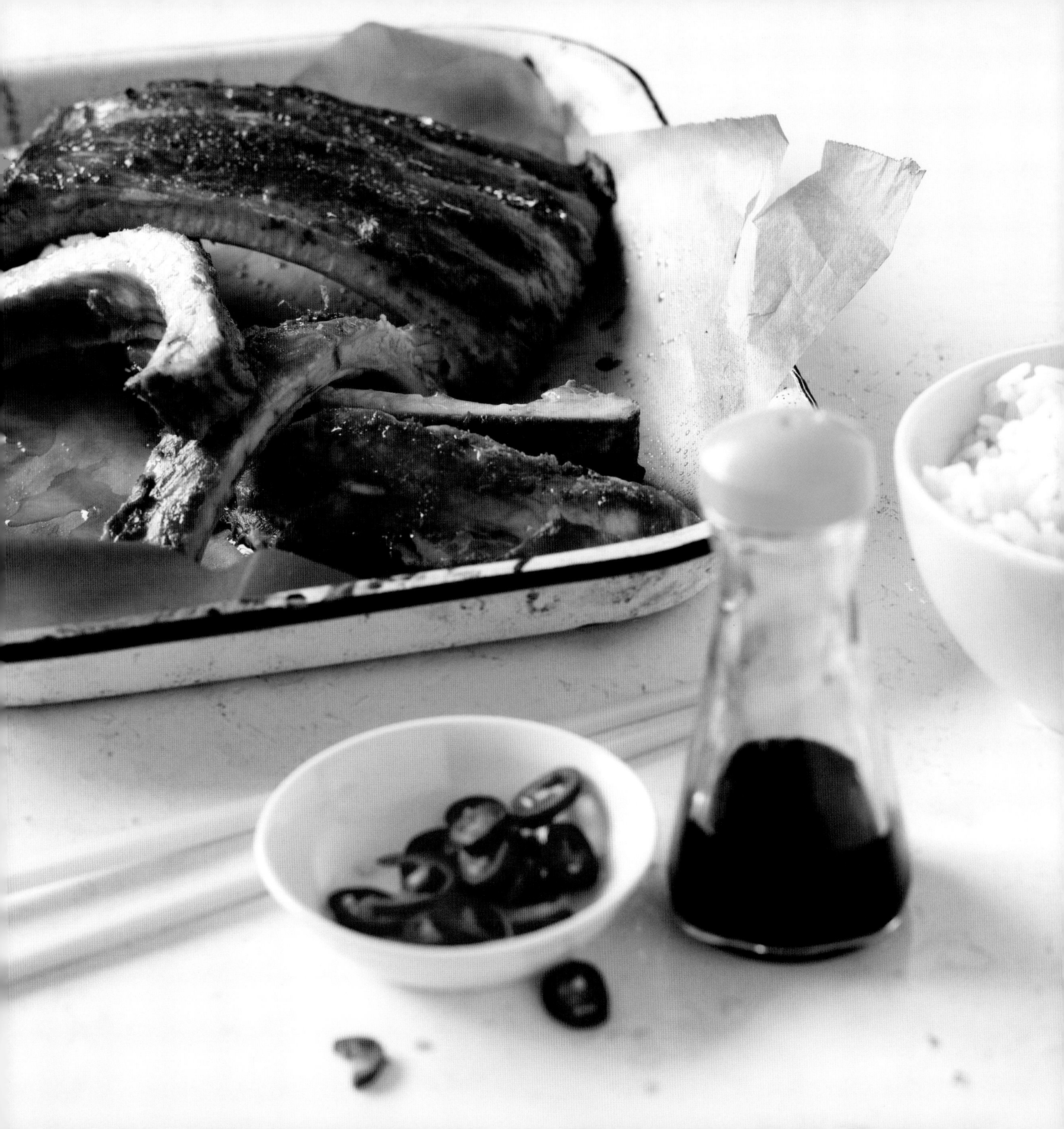

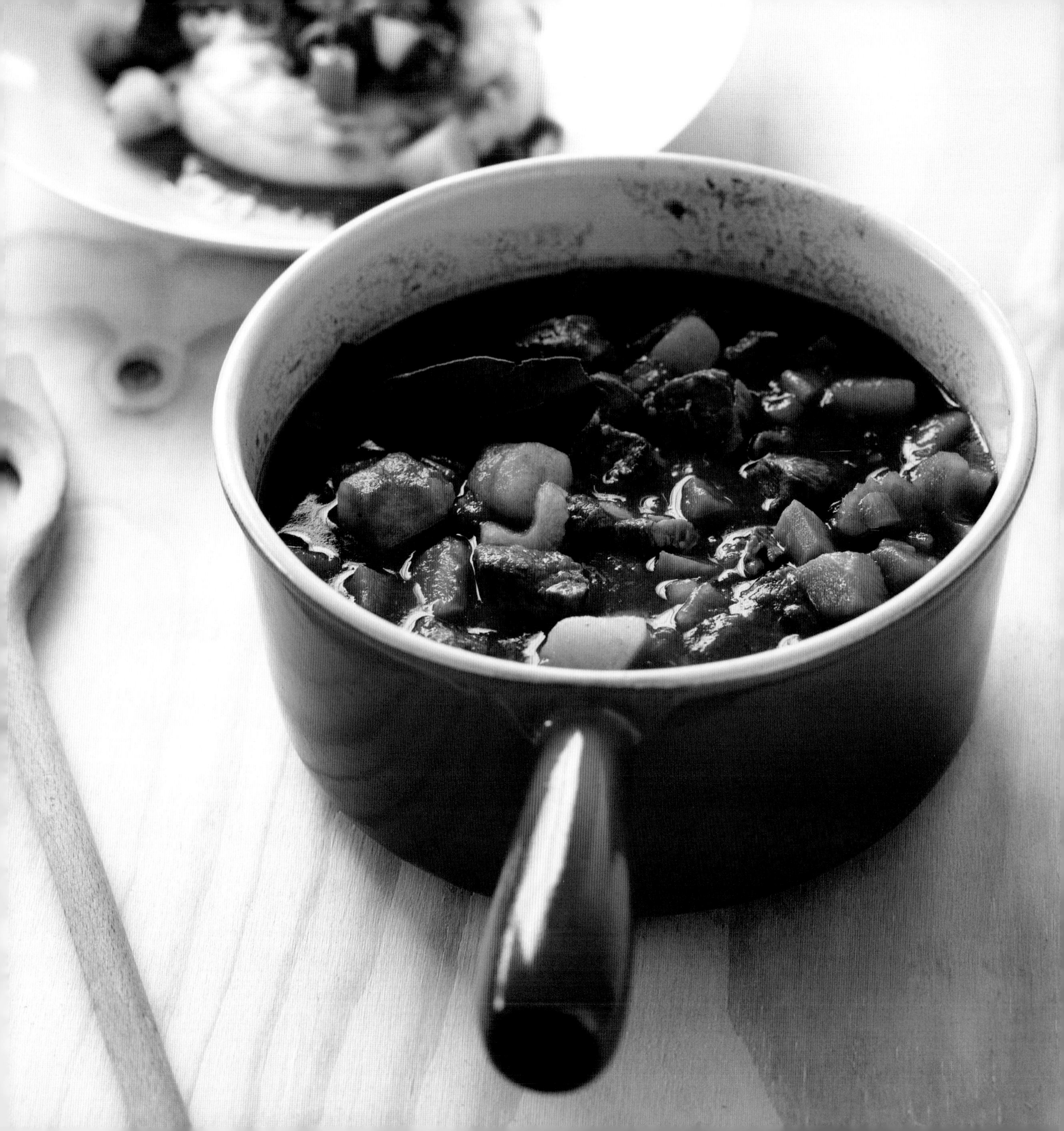

Lamb and vegetable stew

Stews and casseroles are real winners for children, and convenient for busy parents as they are so easy to make. This one is packed with a generous serve of lamb and nutritious vegetables. SERVES 4

2 tablespoons olive oil
1 kg lean stewing lamb, cut into 3 cm cubes
1 onion, diced
3 sticks celery, finely sliced
2 cloves garlic, crushed
3 cups (750 ml) gluten-free, wheat-free, dairy-free, soy-free beef stock
3 cups (750 ml) pureed tomatoes
2 tablespoons tomato paste (puree)
2 bay leaves
2 sprigs of rosemary
salt and freshly ground black pepper
600 g potatoes, cut into chunks
3 carrots, diced
3 tablespoons chopped flat-leaf parsley (optional)
mashed potato or garlic and rosemary polenta (see page 64), to serve

Heat the olive oil in a large stockpot over medium heat, add the lamb and cook for 2–3 minutes until lightly browned. Add the onion, celery and garlic and cook, stirring, for 5 minutes or until the onion has softened.

Reduce the heat to medium–low and stir in the stock, pureed tomatoes, tomato paste, bay leaves and rosemary. Season with salt and pepper, then cover and simmer gently for 2 hours. Add the potato and carrot and simmer for another hour or until the vegetables are tender.

Sprinkle the parsley over the top (if using) and serve with mashed potato or polenta.

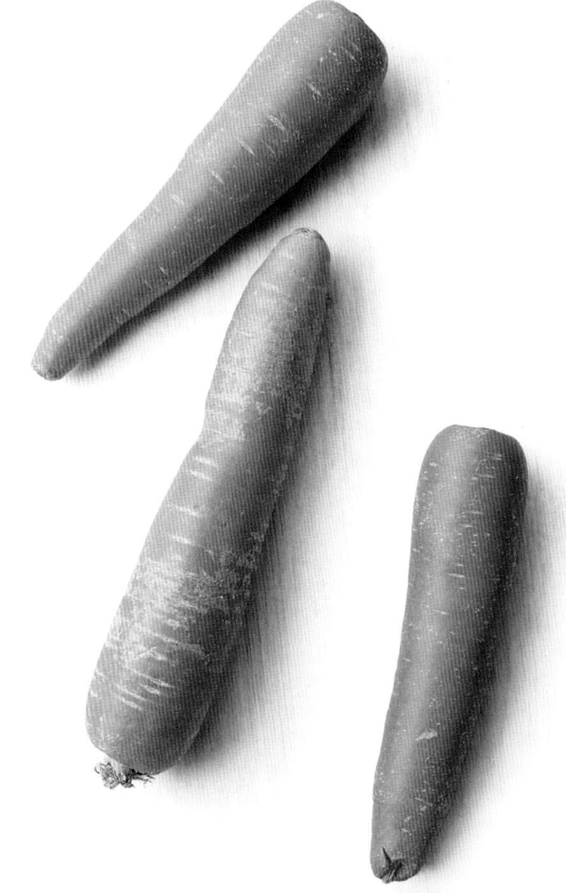

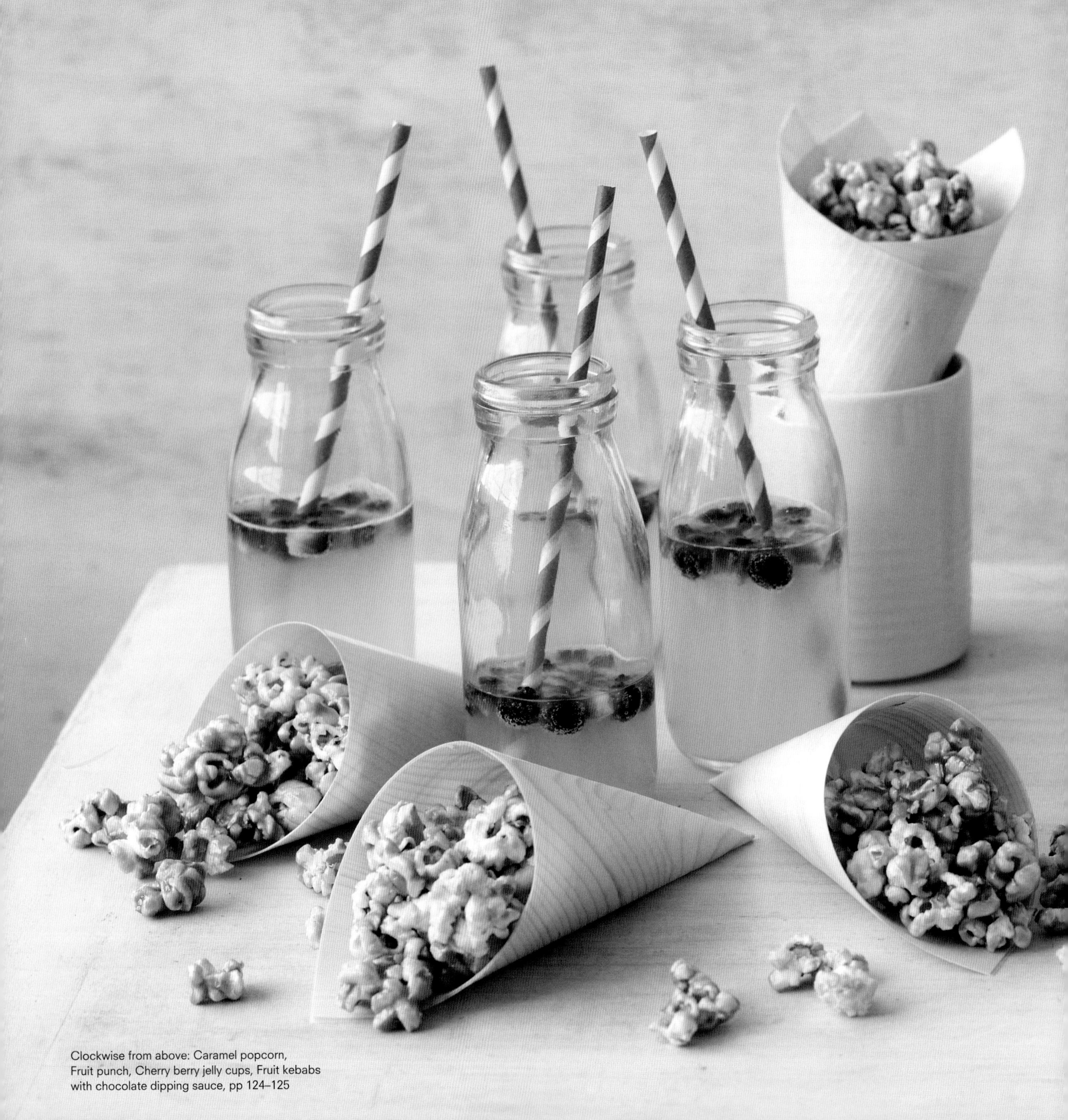

Clockwise from above: Caramel popcorn, Fruit punch, Cherry berry jelly cups, Fruit kebabs with chocolate dipping sauce, pp 124–125

sweet treats for kids

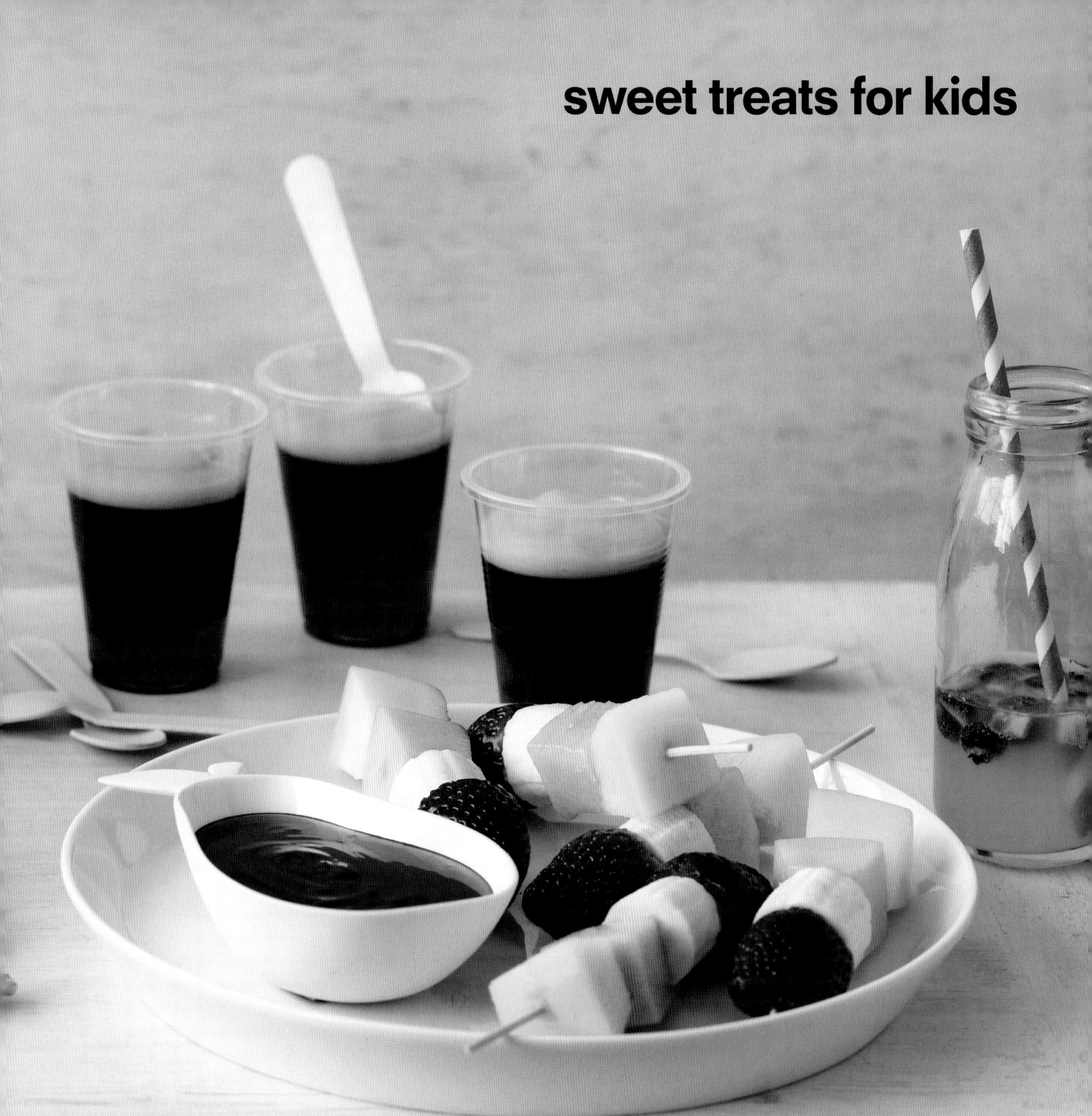

Cherry berry jelly cups

Fruit set in jelly never tasted better than with these little cups, topped with creamy custard. SERVES 8

1 × 85 g packet strawberry jelly crystals
about 3 cups (750 ml) boiling water
150 g strawberries, hulled and chopped
1 × 420 g tin pitted cherries, drained and cut in half (reserve the liquid)
1 tablespoon powdered gelatine
2 tablespoons sugar

CUSTARD TOPPING
2 tablespoons gluten-free, wheat-free, dairy-free, egg-free custard powder
1¼ cups (310 ml) rice milk
2 teaspoons caster sugar

Pour the jelly crystals into a bowl, add 400 ml boiling water and stir until completely dissolved. Set aside to cool slightly. Divide the strawberry pieces among eight ½ cup (125 ml) jelly moulds, then pour the jelly over the top – the moulds should be about half full. Allow to cool to room temperature, then place in the fridge for an hour or so to set firm.

Meanwhile, heat the reserved cherry liquid in a small saucepan over medium–high heat. Dissolve the gelatine in a small amount of boiling water and add to the cherry liquid, along with the sugar and enough boiling water to make a total volume of 350 ml. Cool to room temperature.

Remove the strawberry jelly from the fridge when fully set. Scatter the cherry pieces over the strawberry jelly, then pour the cherry jelly over the top. Place in the fridge for about 2 hours to set firm.

To make the custard topping, blend the custard powder with 3 tablespoons rice milk to make a paste. Heat the remaining rice milk and sugar in a small saucepan until nearly boiling. Slowly add the custard paste, stirring until smooth, and simmer for 1–2 minutes. Cool completely, then spoon over the set jellies. Chill until ready to serve.

Fruit punch

Fizzy fruit punch is always popular at festive gatherings. The quantities given can easily be reduced to enjoy any time. SERVES ABOUT 20

1 litre apple juice
1 litre pineapple juice
1 × 170 g tin passionfruit pulp in syrup
2.5 litres soda water
250 g strawberries, hulled and chopped
125 g blueberries
mint leaves, to taste
ice cubes, to serve

Combine all the ingredients in a large punch bowl. Serve in tall glasses with ice.

Caramel popcorn

You can also make this moreish treat into bars. Simply press the warm mixture into a shallow baking dish lined with baking paper, then place in the fridge until set firm. Cut into bars with a sharp knife. SERVES 8–12

2½ tablespoons soy-free, dairy-free spread
2½ tablespoons copha
½ cup (110 g) brown sugar
3 tablespoons honey
4 cups (50 g) cooked popcorn

Melt the dairy-free spread and copha in a large saucepan over medium heat. Add the brown sugar and honey and stir until the sugar has dissolved. Reduce the heat to medium–low and simmer for 5 minutes or until the sauce has caramelised. Leave to cool slightly.

Place the popcorn in a large mixing bowl. Pour the sauce over the top and stir well to coat and cool (this will stop the popcorn sticking together in large clumps). Serve as is, or make into bars.

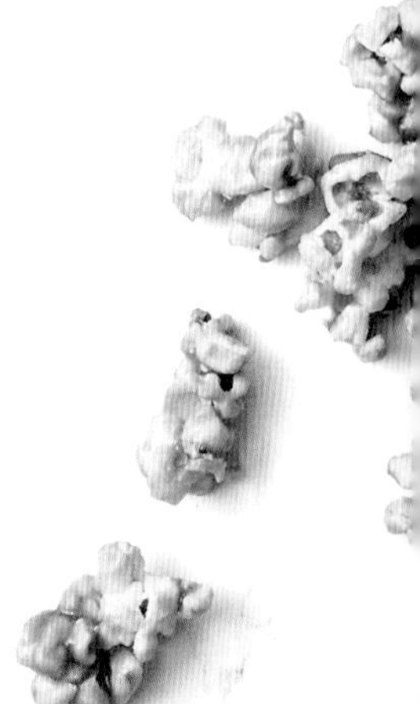

Fruit kebabs with chocolate dipping sauce

Fruit skewers with seasonal fruit make a nutritious sweet treat for kids. A little dip into some allergen-friendly chocolate will ensure the kids will line up for more. MAKES 16

100 g dark gluten-free, wheat-free, dairy-free, nut-free, soy-free chocolate
½ rockmelon, cut into 2 cm cubes
½ honeydew melon, cut into 2 cm cubes
4 bananas, cut into 2 cm chunks
16 small strawberries, hulled

Place the chocolate in a small glass bowl set over a saucepan of simmering water (make sure the base of the bowl does not touch the water) and stir until melted.

Thread one piece of honeydew melon, rockmelon and banana onto a small wooden skewer, followed by a strawberry. Repeat with the remaining ingredients to make 16 skewers. Serve with the melted chocolate for dipping.

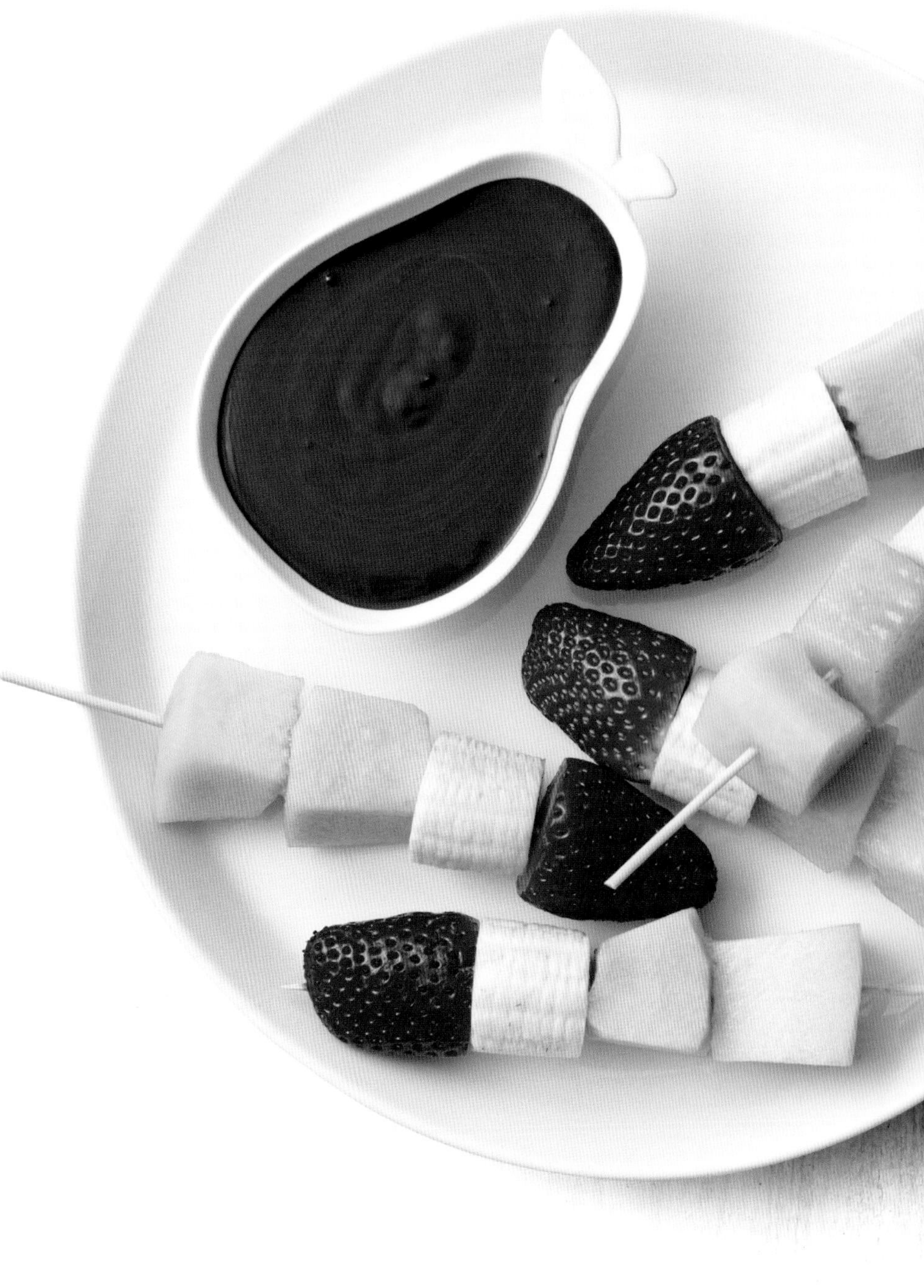

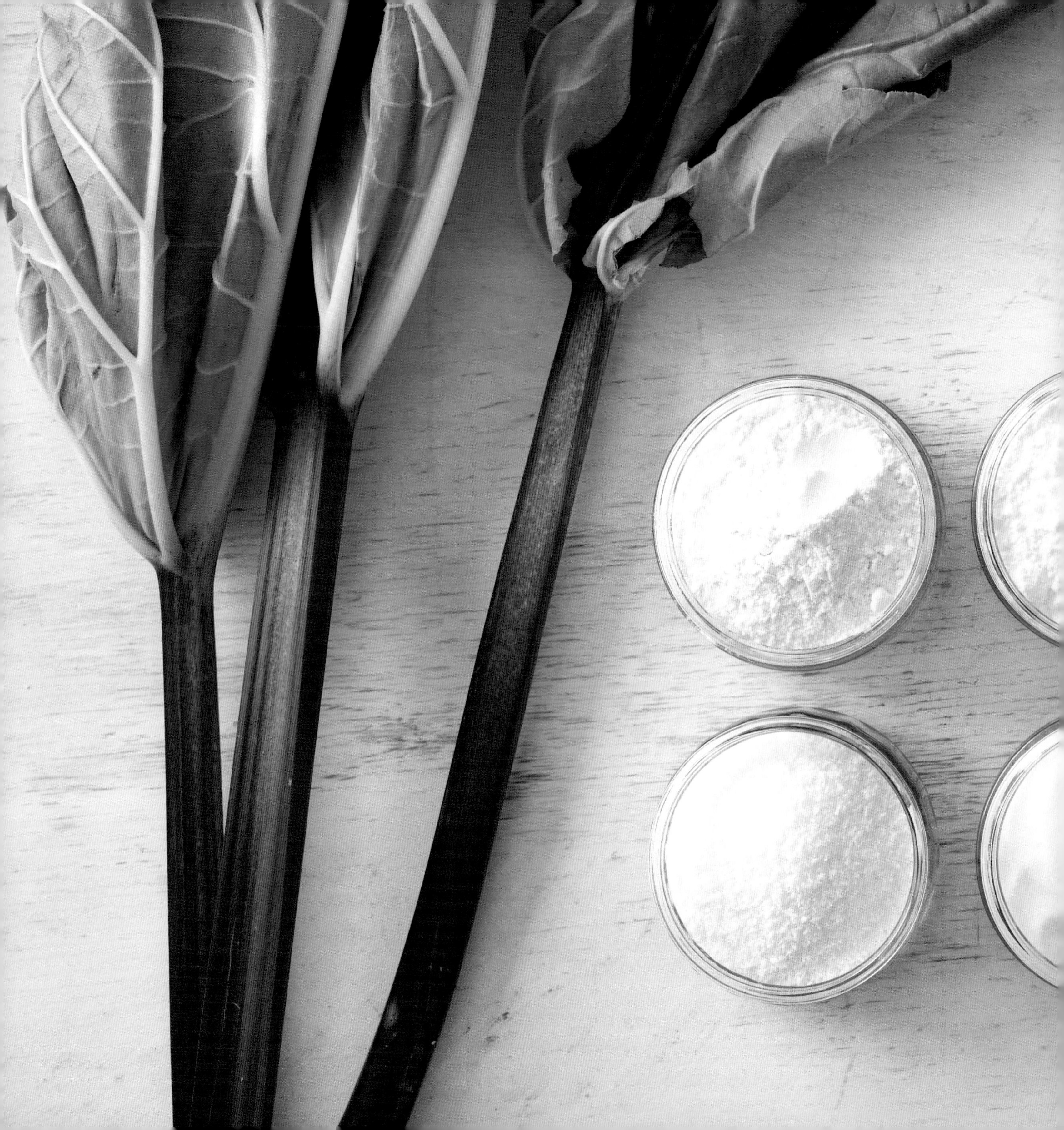

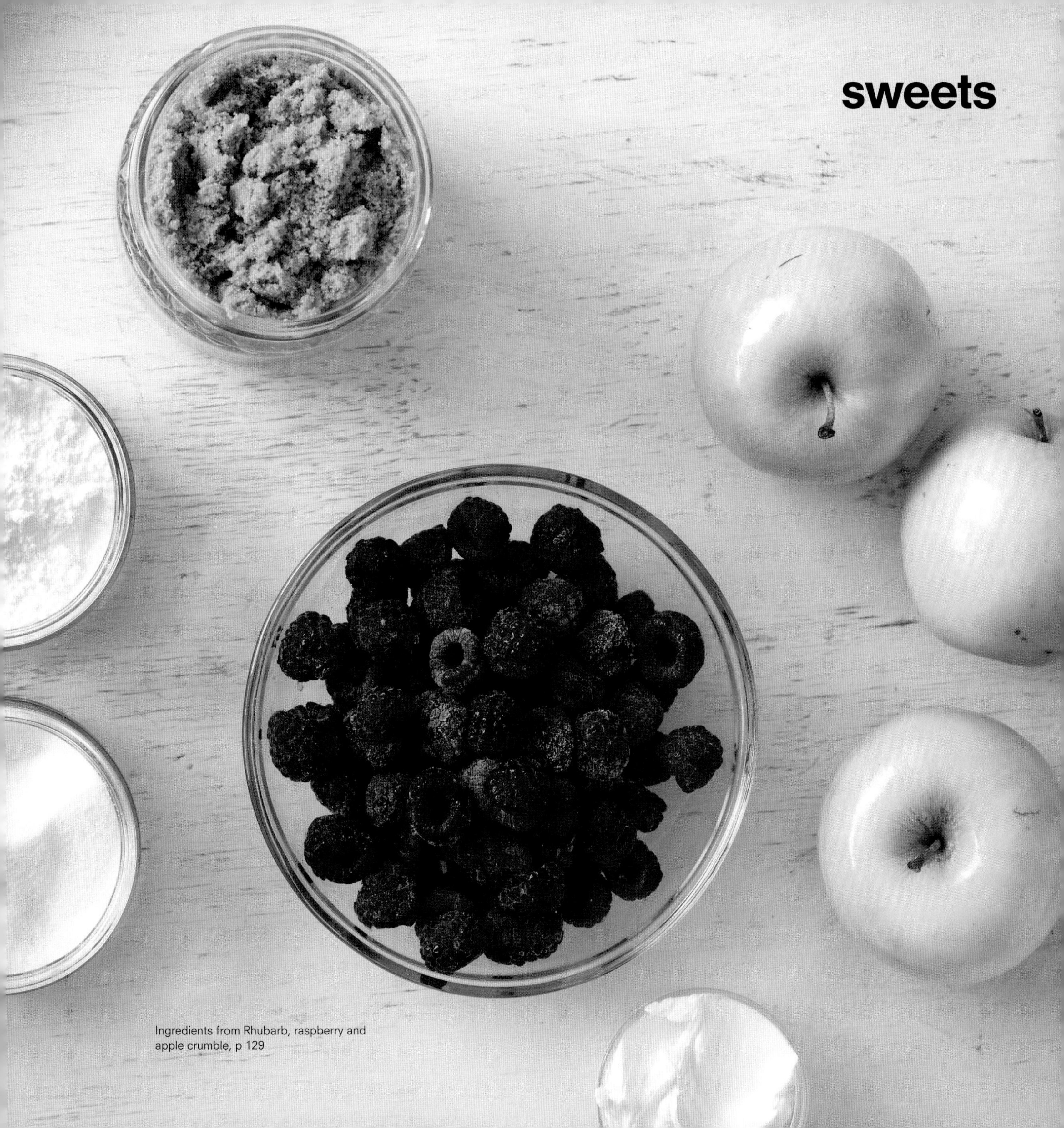

sweets

Ingredients from Rhubarb, raspberry and apple crumble, p 129

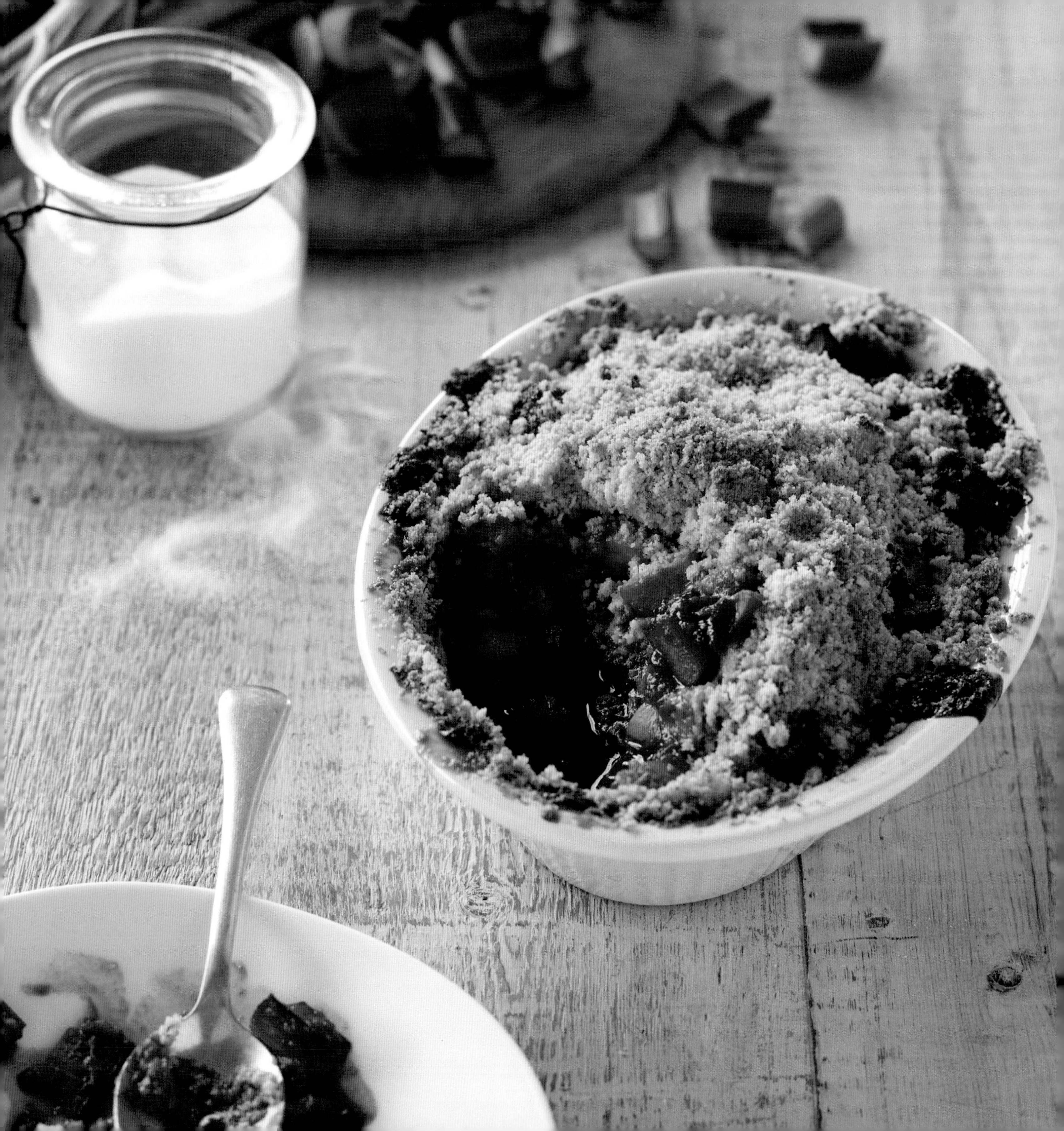

Rhubarb, raspberry and apple crumble

I love fruit crumbles but they often have wheat and oat toppings, which makes them off limits for many of us. This recipe is a delight as it contains no allergens. It can be enjoyed warm or cold and is especially good served with allergen-free custard. If you are allergic to coconut, leave it out of the recipe – it will still taste great! SERVES 6

1 bunch rhubarb, stalks trimmed and cut into 1.5 cm pieces
4 apples, peeled, cored and diced
½ cup (110 g) sugar
1 × 400 g tin raspberries in syrup, drained (or use fresh, if preferred)
3 tablespoons pure icing sugar
1½ cups (195 g) fine rice flour
1 cup (220 g) brown sugar
⅓ cup (25 g) desiccated coconut
120 g soy-free, dairy-free spread, at room temperature

Preheat the oven to 180°C and lightly grease a medium baking dish.

Place the rhubarb, apple, sugar and 1.5 litres water in a medium saucepan over medium–high heat. Bring to the boil, then reduce the heat and simmer for 6–8 minutes or until just tender. Drain.

Combine the rhubarb mixture, raspberries and icing sugar in a bowl, then spoon into the baking dish.

Place the flour, brown sugar and coconut in a medium bowl and rub in the spread until the mixture resembles fine breadcrumbs. Sprinkle evenly over the fruit mixture and bake for 30 minutes or until golden brown.

Passionfruit puddings

These passionfruit puddings set like mini mousses. They are light and zesty, and are made with coconut cream for a really creamy texture. Coconut milk will not give the same result so I'd advise against using it as a substitute. This recipe is unsuitable if you are allergic to coconut – if you have no issue with dairy, replace the coconut cream with cream. SERVES 4

1 × 85 g packet passionfruit jelly crystals
200 ml boiling water
200 ml coconut cream, chilled
pulp from 1 passionfruit
1 × 170 g tin passionfruit pulp in syrup

Pour the jelly crystals into a large bowl, add the boiling water and stir until completely dissolved. Set aside to cool to room temperature.

Place the bowl over a larger bowl filled with ice cubes. Pour in the chilled coconut cream and beat with hand-held electric beaters on high until the mixture doubles in volume. Fold in the passionfruit pulp. Pour into four ½ cup (125 ml) ramekins or bowls and place in the fridge for an hour or so until set.

Just before serving, drizzle a little passionfruit pulp in syrup over each pudding.

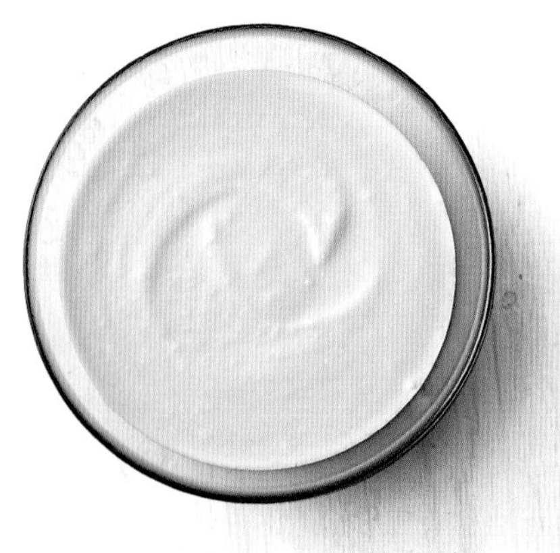

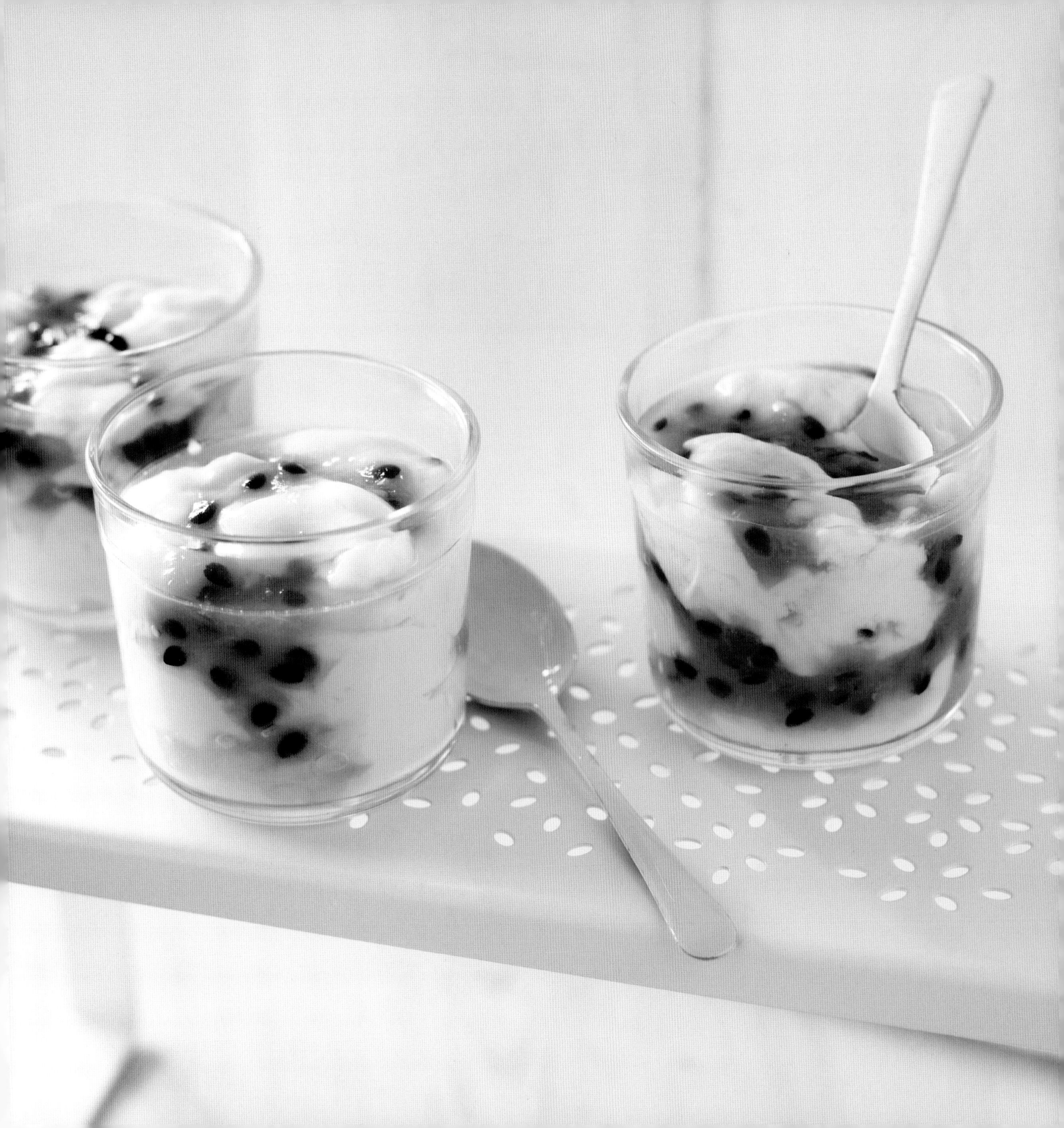

Chocolate pancakes with caramel sauce

Everyone loves pancakes! This recipe makes a really decadent dessert, bringing together the much-loved combination of caramel and chocolate. SERVES 4

⅔ cup (85 g) fine rice flour
3 tablespoons besan flour
⅓ cup (50 g) maize cornflour
¾ teaspoon gluten-free baking powder
2 tablespoons cocoa powder
2½ tablespoons sugar
1 egg*
175 ml rice milk
1 tablespoon soy-free, dairy-free spread, melted, plus extra to serve (optional)
cooking spray

CARAMEL SAUCE
2 tablespoons soy-free, dairy-free spread
100 g brown sugar
2 tablespoons rice milk

Sift the flours, baking powder and cocoa powder into a large bowl and add the sugar. Combine the egg and milk in a bowl, then pour into the dry ingredients and mix with a spoon until well combined. Stir in the melted spread, then leave the batter to rest for 10 minutes.

Place a large frying pan over low–medium heat for a minute or two. When hot, lightly spray with cooking spray, then add 2–3 tablespoons of batter per pancake. Cook for 2–3 minutes or until bubbles start to appear, then flip over and cook the other side for 2 minutes. Remove and keep warm while you make the remaining pancakes (you should have enough batter to make eight).

To make the caramel sauce, melt the spread in a small saucepan over medium–low heat. Add the brown sugar and rice milk and cook for about 2–3 minutes or until the sugar has dissolved and the sauce has started to caramelise.

Divide the pancakes among four plates, top with a little extra spread (if using), then pour over the sauce and serve.

***For egg allergy**
Place 1 teaspoon psyllium husks in a small bowl and pour over 3 tablespoons boiling water, stirring constantly to ensure the psyllium does not clump together. Set aside for 4–5 minutes until it forms a gel, stirring occasionally. Use in place of the egg.

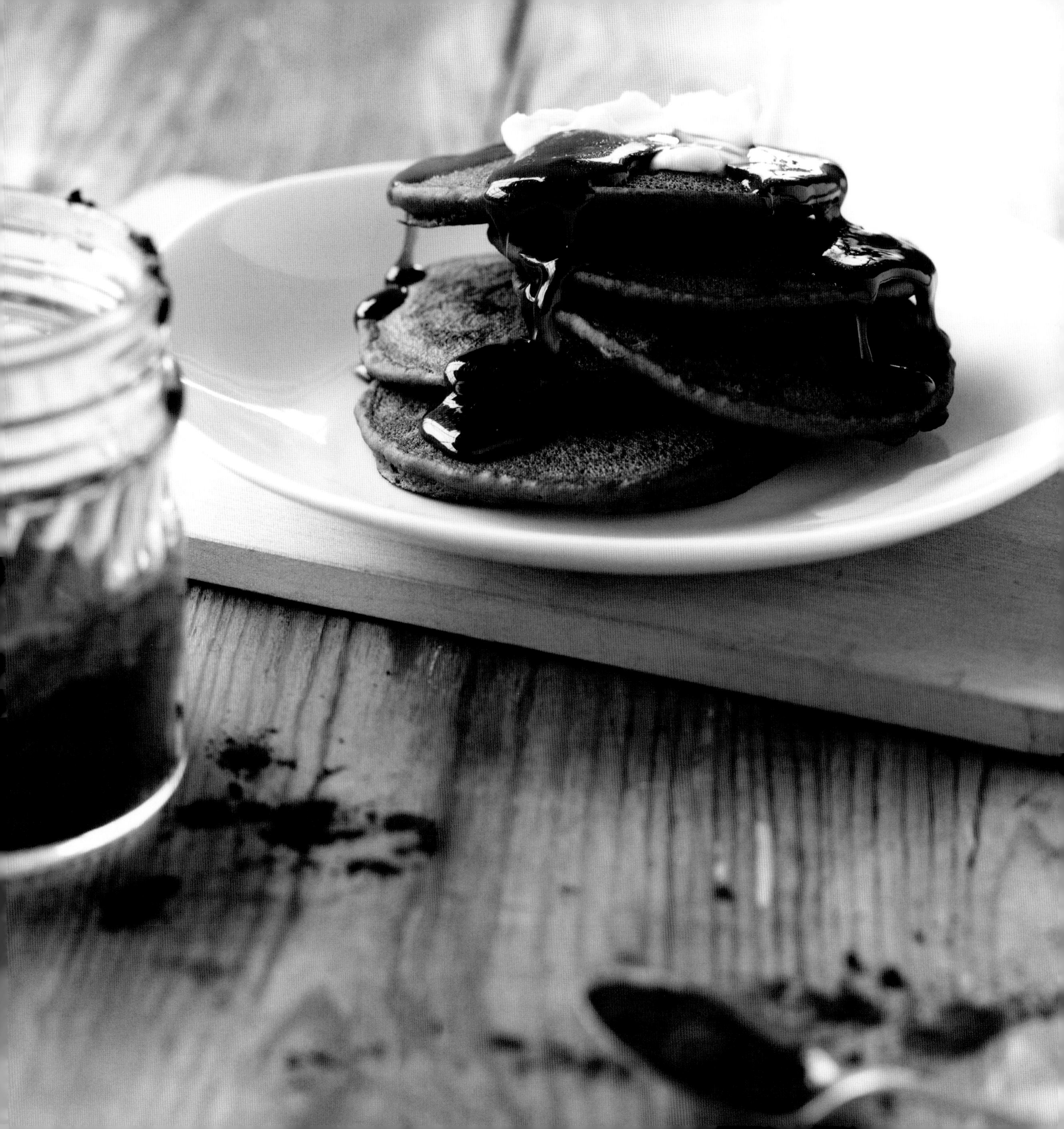

Choc-orange mousse

Normally chocolate mousse is full of dairy and eggs. This version is allergy free, using avocados as a creamy base. This may seem like an unusual ingredient in a dessert, but trust me – you'll love it. SERVES 4

2 ripe avocados
3 teaspoons vanilla essence
½ cup (50 g) cocoa powder
1 cup (160 g) pure icing sugar
1 tablespoon finely grated orange zest
fresh berries and mint leaves, to serve

Cut the avocados in half and scoop out flesh. Place in a food processor with the vanilla, cocoa, icing sugar and orange zest and process until smooth and well combined.

Spoon the mixture into four bowls or glasses and refrigerate for 1 hour. Decorate with fresh berries and mint leaves just before serving.

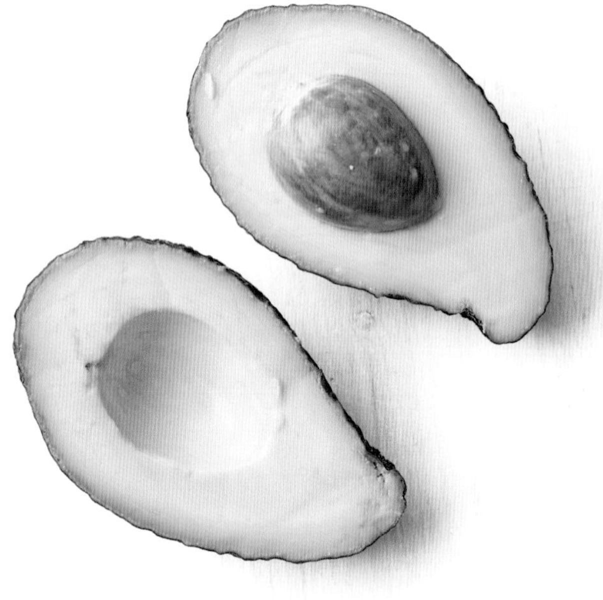

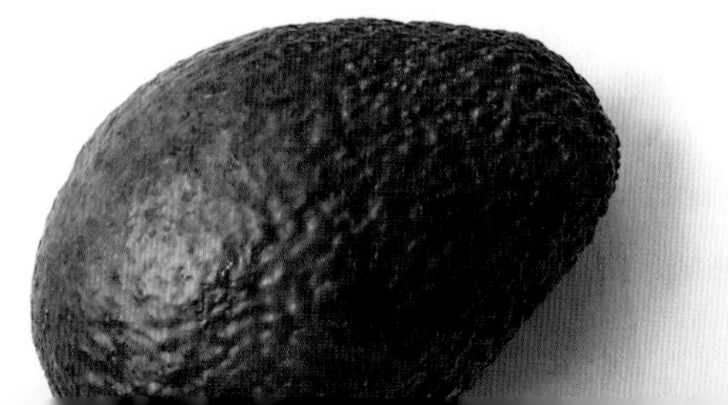

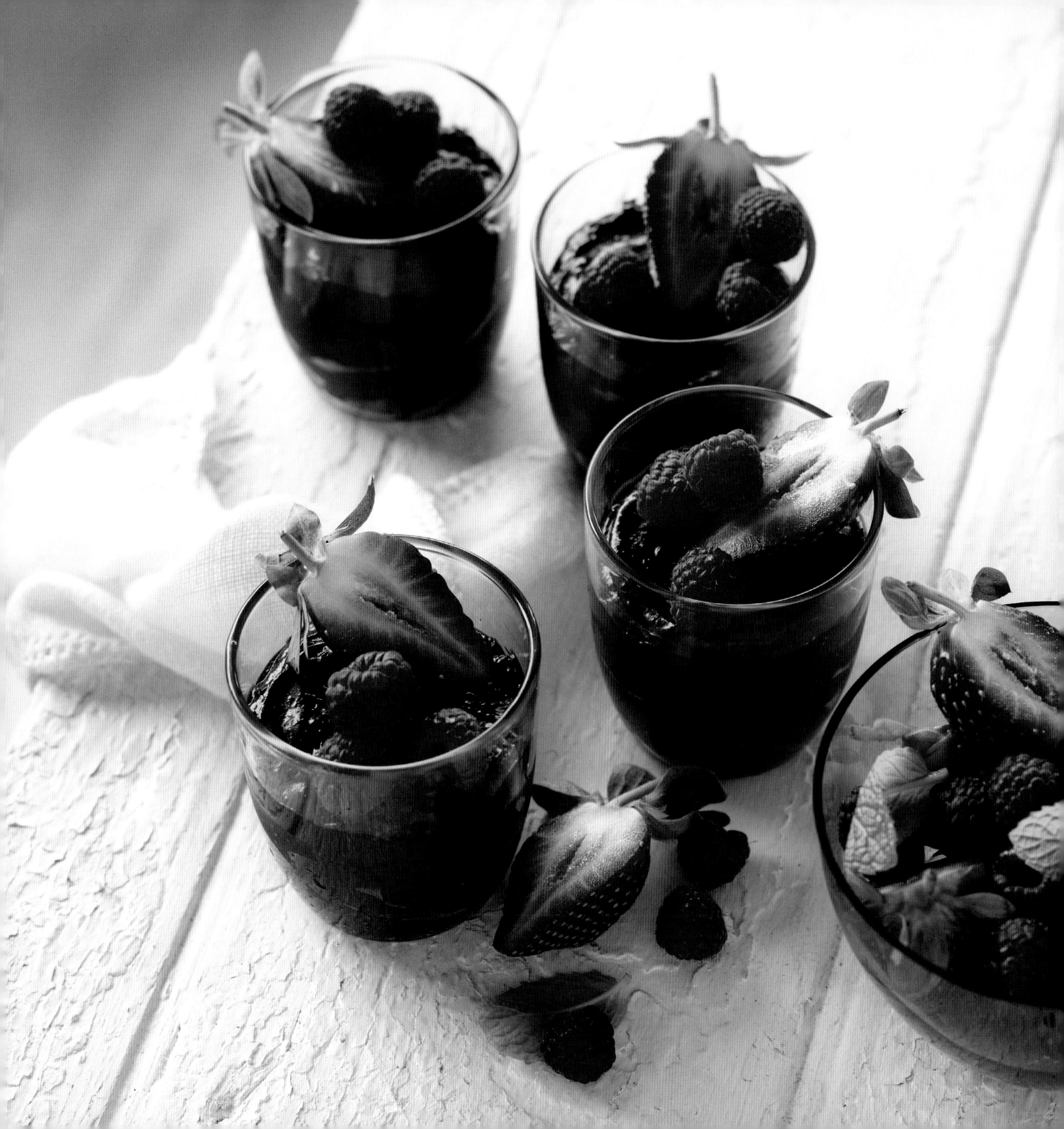

Jamaican apple tart

This apple tart is a little bit different, made with sultanas and bananas cooked in a caramel sauce. The rum and lemon zest add an extra element of surprise. It tastes fabulous! If you don't have time to make the pastry, allergy-friendly pastry sheets can be found in the freezer section of health-food shops and some supermarkets.

SERVES 6–8

½ cup (80 g) sultanas
3 tablespoons dark rum
3 tablespoons caster sugar
4 granny smith apples, peeled and thinly sliced
2 tablespoons soy-free, dairy-free spread
3 tablespoons brown sugar, plus extra for sprinkling
grated zest and juice of 1 lemon
3 bananas, sliced

GLUTEN-FREE, WHEAT-FREE, DAIRY-FREE, EGG-FREE, NUT-FREE, SOY-FREE PASTRY
1 cup (130 g) fine rice flour
½ cup (75 g) maize cornflour
½ cup (45 g) besan flour
1 teaspoon xanthan gum
3 tablespoons caster sugar
160 g soy-free, dairy-free spread
4 tablespoons iced water

Place the sultanas and rum in a small bowl and stir well to combine. Set aside to soak for an hour.

To make the pastry, sift the flours and xanthan gum into a bowl. Transfer to a food processor, add the sugar and spread and process until the mixture resembles fine breadcrumbs. With the motor running, add the iced water (a tablespoon at a time) to form a soft dough. Turn out onto a bench dusted with gluten-free, wheat-free cornflour and knead until smooth. Wrap in plastic film and refrigerate for 30 minutes. Place the dough between two sheets of baking paper and roll out to a thickness of 3–5 mm.

Preheat the oven to 170°C. Grease a rectangular fluted tart dish (mine is 11 cm × 40 cm).

Ease the pastry into the tart dish and trim the edges. Line the pastry case with baking paper, fill with baking beads or rice and blind-bake for 10–15 minutes or until lightly golden. Remove the paper and beads or rice and set aside to cool.

Bring a medium saucepan of water to the boil. Add the caster sugar and stir to dissolve, then add the apple slices and simmer over medium–low heat for 2 minutes or until tender. Drain.

Place the spread, brown sugar, lemon zest and juice in a large frying pan over medium–low heat until melted and combined. Add the apple, banana and sultana and rum mixture and stir to combine. Remove the fruit with a slotted spoon and place evenly in the pasty case. Sprinkle a little extra brown sugar over the top and bake for 30–35 minutes or until the pastry is a deep golden brown and the filling is cooked through and syrupy. Allow to sit for 10 minutes before serving.

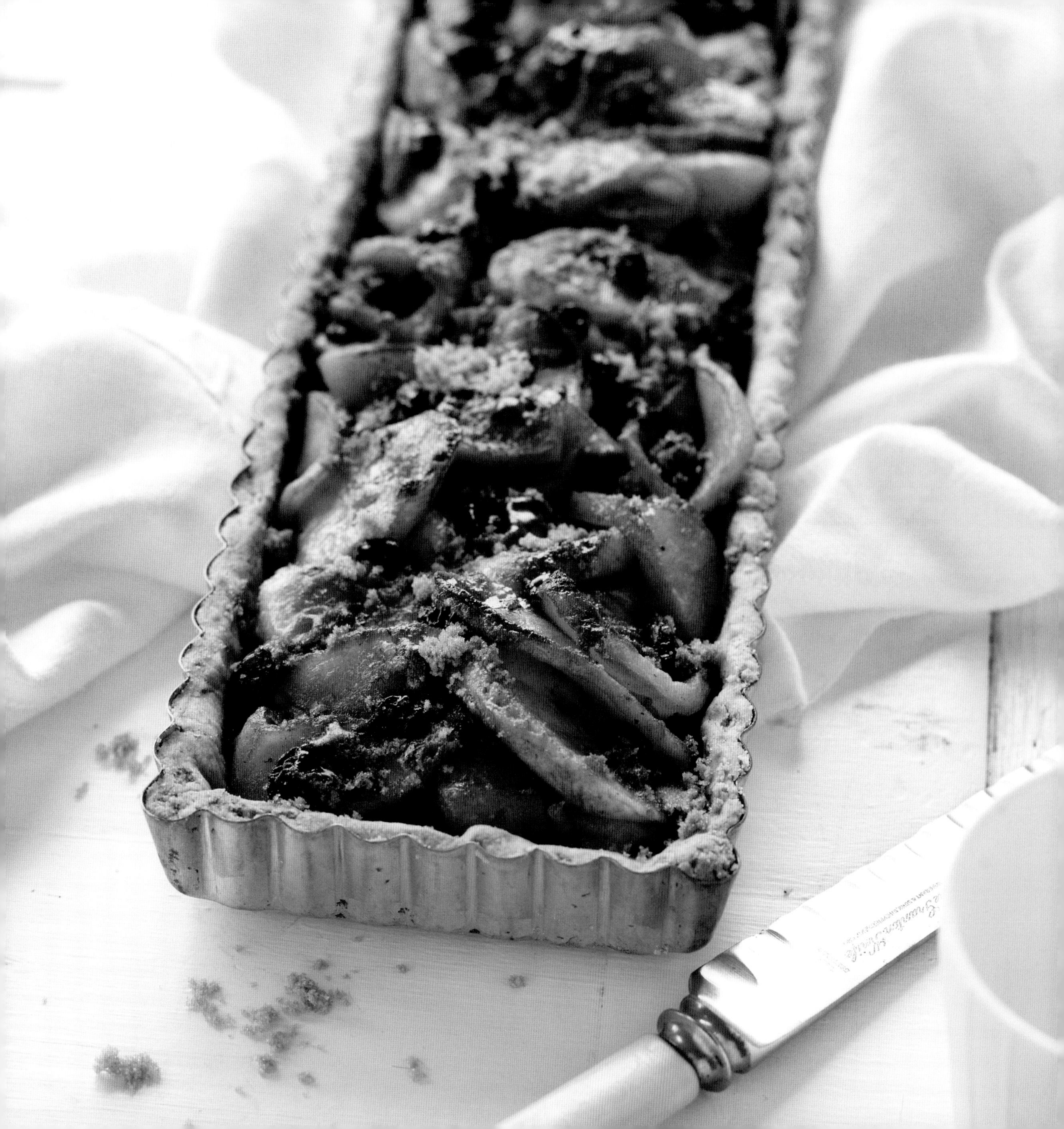

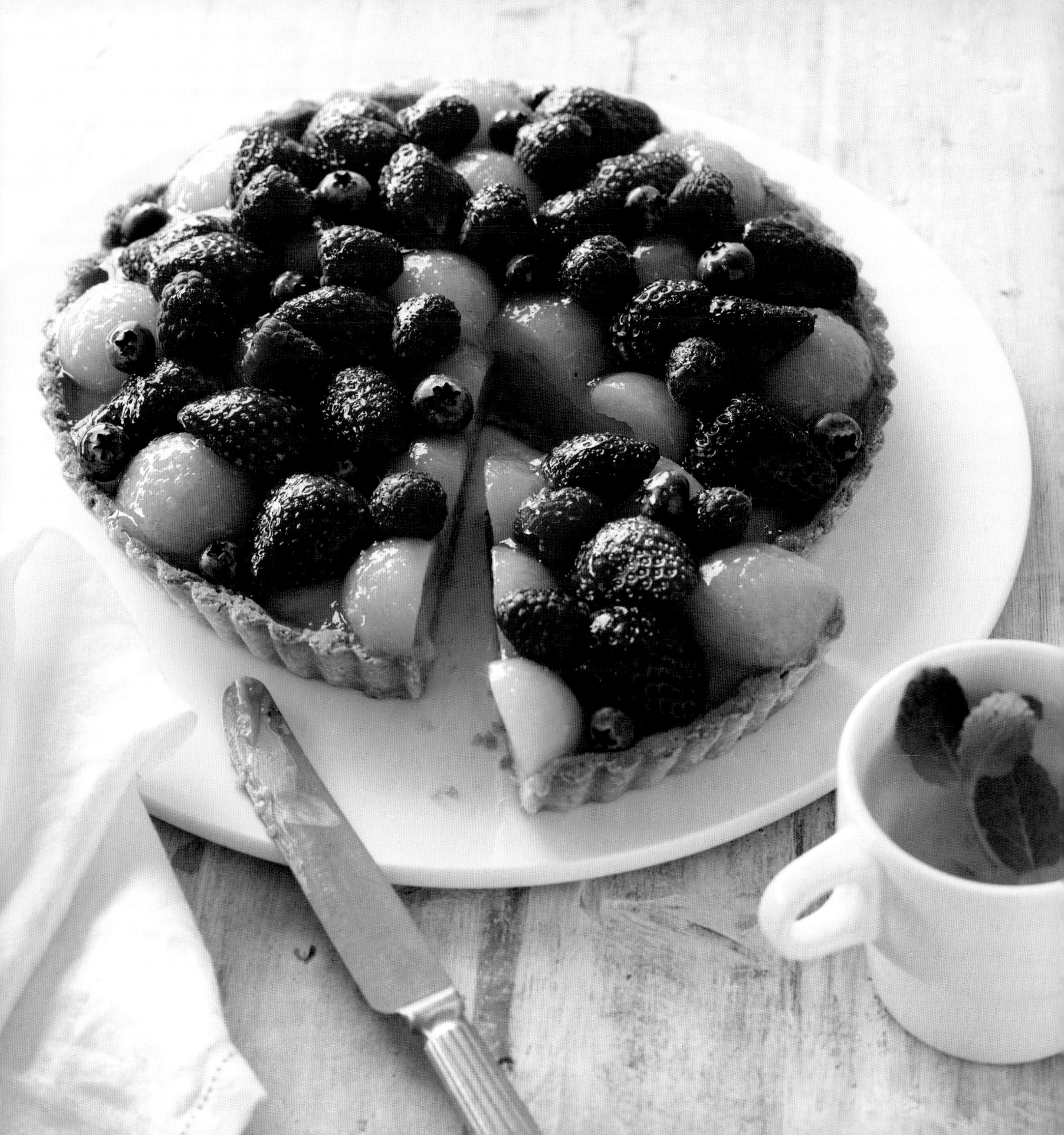

Fruit custard flan

This recipe uses ready-made allergy-friendly pastry, which can be purchased frozen at specialty health-food shops and some larger supermarkets. Alternatively, make your own pastry, following the recipe on page 136. You can top the custard with any fruit you like – the selection given here is just a suggestion. SERVES 8–10

1 sheet gluten-free, wheat-free, dairy-free, soy-free, sweet shortcrust pastry*
1 × 85 g packet pineapple jelly crystals
140 g tinned apricot halves, drained
250 g strawberries, hulled and larger ones cut in half
75 g raspberries
75 g blueberries

CUSTARD FILLING
¾ cup (90 g) gluten-free, wheat-free, dairy-free custard powder*
3 cups (750 ml) rice milk
3 tablespoons caster sugar
2 teaspoons vanilla essence

Preheat the oven to 170°C. Grease a 23 cm fluted flan tin.

Place the pastry in the tin and trim the edges. Line the pastry case with baking paper, fill with baking beads or rice and blind-bake for 10–15 minutes or until lightly golden. Remove the paper and beads or rice and set aside to cool.

Meanwhile, to make the custard filling, blend the custard powder with 2 tablespoons of the rice milk to form a smooth paste. Combine the sugar and remaining milk in a medium saucepan over medium–high heat and bring almost to the boil. Reduce the heat to low, then add the custard paste and vanilla and stir until well combined and the custard is very thick. Pour into the pastry case and chill in the fridge for 1 hour.

In a heatproof jug, prepare the jelly according to the packet directions but use only half the quantity of water. Set aside in the fridge until just starting to set.

Remove the flan from the fridge. Arrange the apricot halves over the custard, followed by the strawberries, raspberries and blueberries.

Slowly pour the pineapple jelly over the fruit to cover in a thin layer and fill the spaces between the fruit. Return the flan to the fridge and leave to chill and set for 2–3 hours before serving.

***For egg allergy**
Make sure you buy egg-free pastry and custard powder.

Self-saucing banana pudding with caramel sauce

This was one of my favourite desserts as a child and I have been working on an allergen-free version for some time. Success at last and I am thrilled with the results. This is extra good served with allergy-friendly custard.

SERVES 6–8

½ cup (65 g) fine rice flour
3 tablespoons maize cornflour
3 tablespoons besan flour
2 teaspoons gluten-free baking powder
1 teaspoon bicarbonate of soda
1 teaspoon xanthan gum
¾ cup (165 g) caster sugar
2 eggs, lightly beaten*
2 ripe bananas, mashed
200 ml rice milk
1 teaspoon vanilla essence
2 tablespoons soy-free, dairy-free spread, melted
⅔ cup (150 g) brown sugar

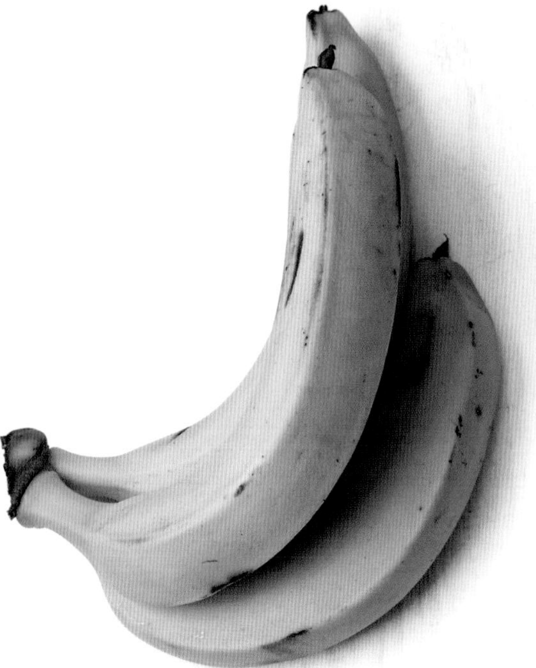

Preheat the oven to 180°C. Lightly grease a 1.5 litre baking dish.

Sift the flours, baking powder, bicarbonate of soda, xanthan gum and caster sugar into a medium bowl.

In a small bowl, combine the egg, mashed banana, rice milk, vanilla and melted spread. Add to the dry ingredients and mix with a wooden spoon until well combined. Pour the mixture into the baking dish.

Combine the brown sugar and 450 ml hot water and pour over the pudding. Bake for 50–60 minutes. Allow to sit for a few minutes before serving.

***For egg allergy**
Place 2 teaspoons psyllium husks in a small bowl and pour over ½ cup (125 ml) boiling water, stirring constantly to ensure the psyllium does not clump together. Set aside for 4–5 minutes until it forms a gel, stirring occasionally. Use in place of the egg.

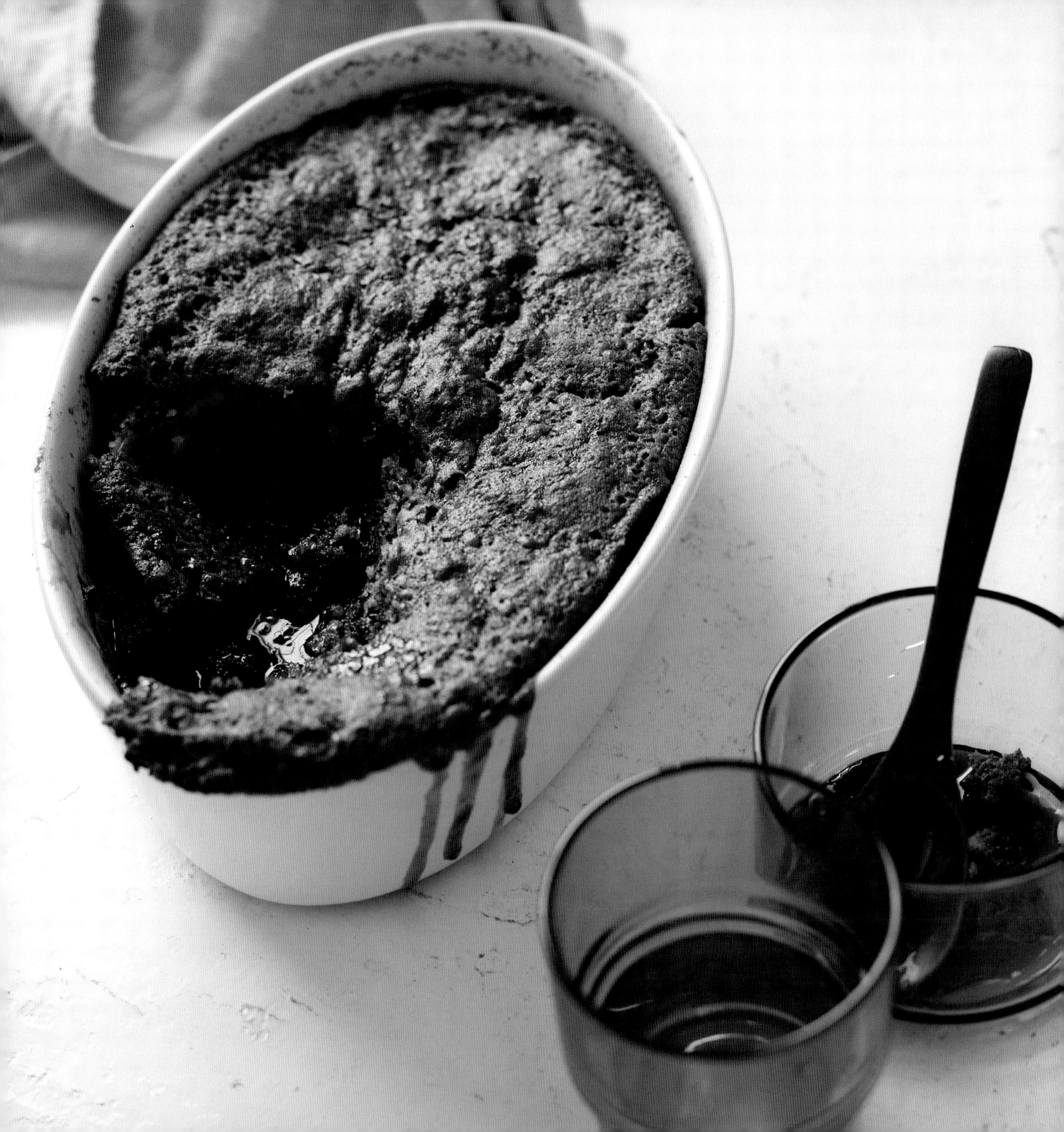

Coconut rice pudding

My sister and I loved this pudding when we were little, and Mum used to make it often. It takes a while to prepare and you need to pay careful attention so you don't burn the rice at the bottom of the pan. This recipe is unsuitable if you are allergic to coconut – if you have no issue with dairy, replace the coconut cream with cream and omit the shredded coconut. SERVES 4

¾ cup (165 g) caster sugar
3 cups (750 ml) rice milk (more if needed)
400 ml light coconut cream
2 teaspoons vanilla essence
1½ cups (300 g) arborio rice
4 tablespoons shredded coconut (optional)
maple syrup, to serve (optional)

Place the sugar, rice milk, coconut cream and vanilla in a medium saucepan over medium–high heat and bring to the boil, stirring regularly. Add the rice. Reduce the heat and simmer, stirring regularly, for about 50 minutes or until the liquid has been absorbed and the rice is tender. Add extra rice milk if required.

Meanwhile, if using the shredded coconut, preheat the oven to 170°C and line a baking tray with foil. Sprinkle the coconut over the tray and bake for 10–12 minutes or until just starting to turn golden brown.

Serve the rice pudding warm or at room temperature topped with toasted coconut and a drizzle of maple syrup (if using).

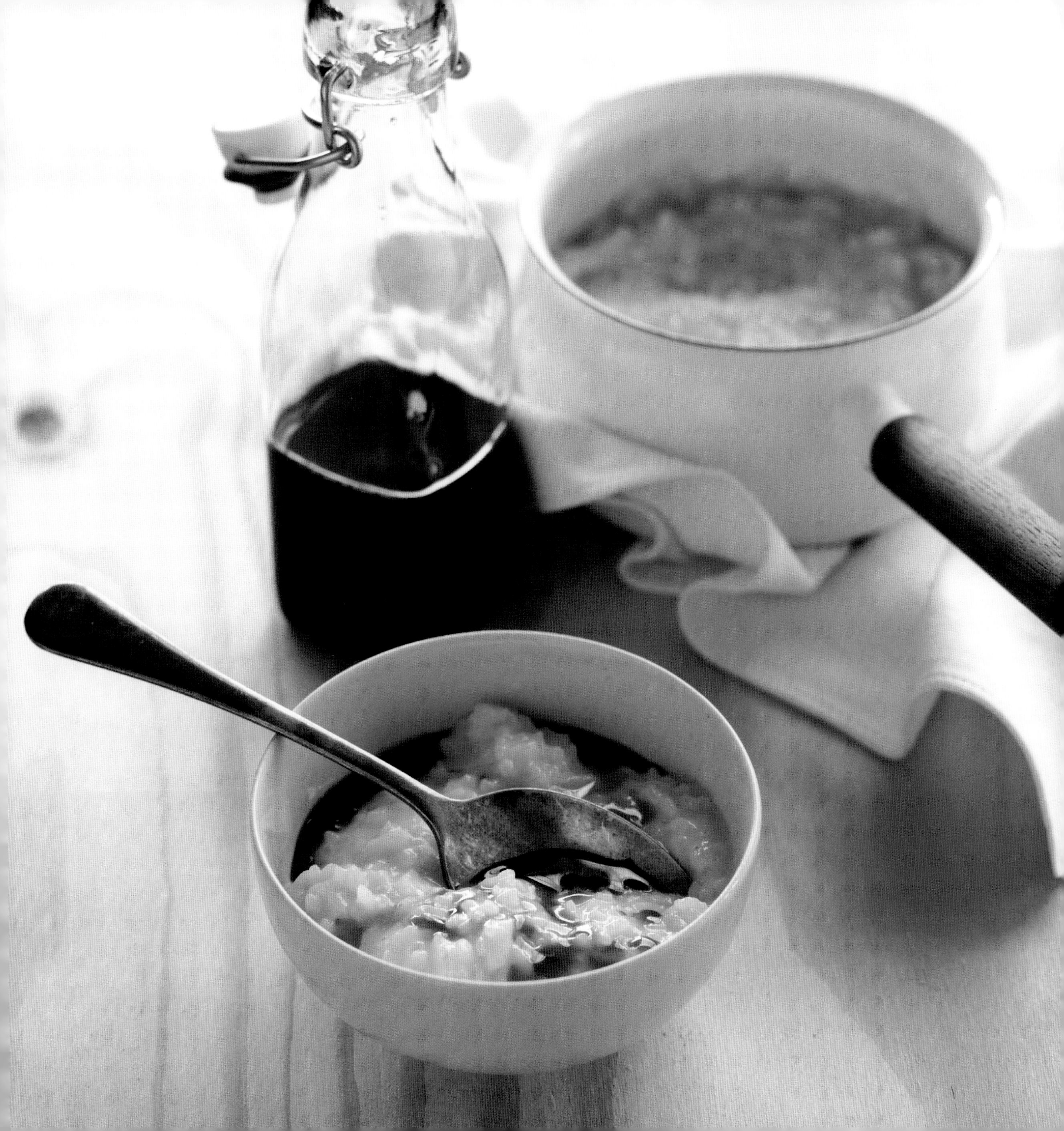

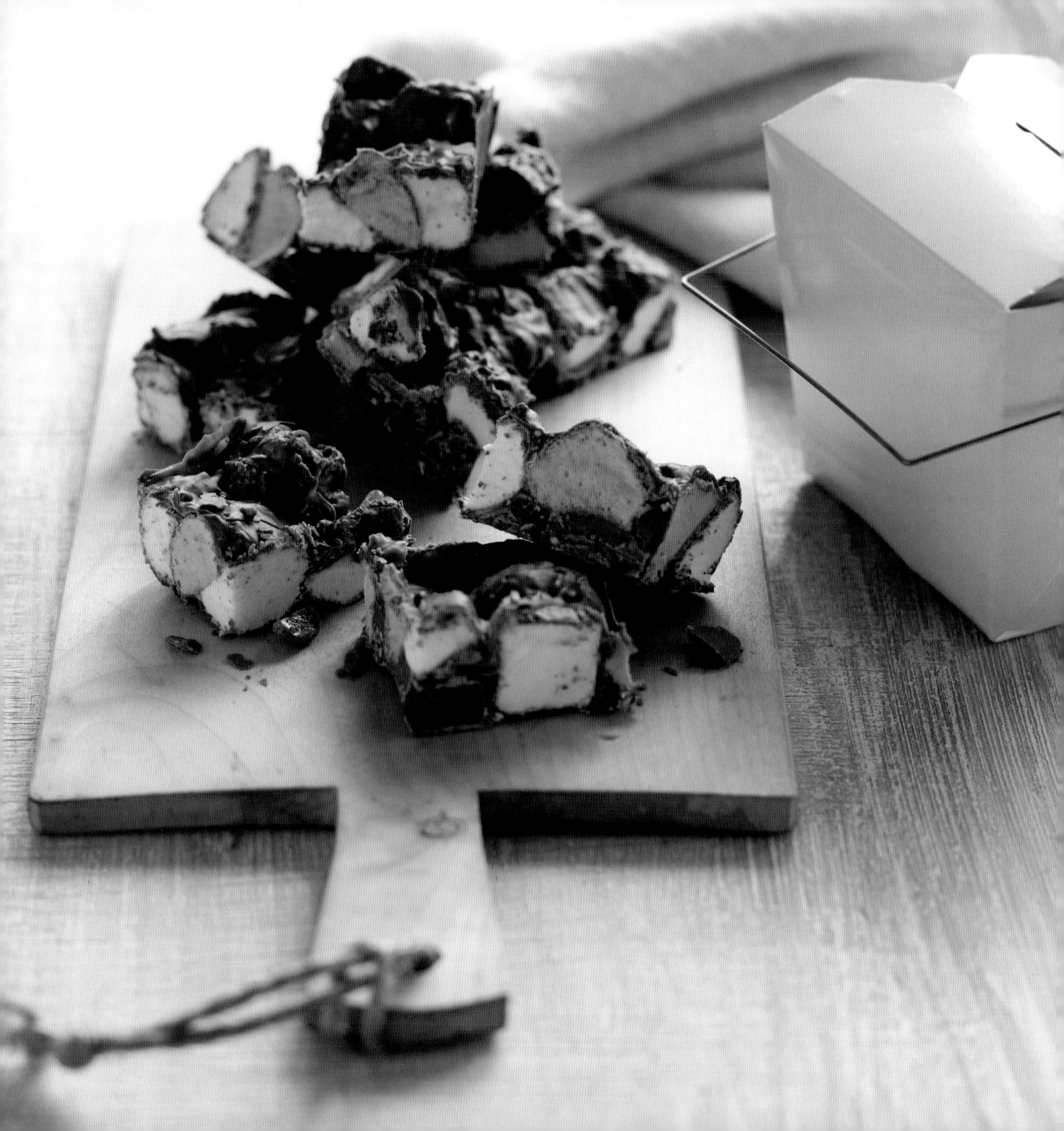

< Rocky road

Many brands of marshmallows and confectionery contain allergens. Make sure you read the labels carefully so you can enjoy this special-occasion treat. Omit the shredded coconut from the recipe if you are allergic to coconut. If you like, you can also make individual serves by spooning the mixture into small paper patty cases.

MAKES ABOUT 20 PIECES

180 g gluten-free, wheat-free, dairy-free, nut-free, soy-free chocolate
3 tablespoons shredded coconut
60 g gluten-free, wheat-free red jelly confectionery (such as red snakes or jelly babies), chopped
110 g gluten-free, wheat-free, dairy-free, soy-free marshmallows, chopped

Line a 17 cm square baking dish with baking paper.

Place the chocolate in a medium glass bowl set over a small saucepan of simmering water (make sure the base of the bowl does not touch the water) and stir until melted.

Combine the remaining ingredients in a large mixing bowl. Pour over the melted chocolate and stir to ensure everything is well mixed and fully coated.

Transfer the rocky road mix to the baking dish and press it to the edges with a metal spoon. Chill in the fridge for 3–4 hours or until firm. Cut into small pieces to serve.

Choc-honey clusters with dried fruit

These clusters are a nice little snack to nibble for morning or afternoon tea. They can also be served on a fruit platter. If you are allergic to coconut, just leave it out of the recipe – the clusters will still be delicious. MAKES 20–25

½ cup (80 g) finely chopped dried apricots
½ cup (80 g) sultanas
1 tablespoon desiccated coconut, plus extra for coating
1 tablespoon honey
50 g gluten-free, wheat-free, dairy-free, nut-free, soy-free dark chocolate
1 teaspoon grated orange zest

Line a baking tray with baking paper.

Combine the dried apricot, sultanas and coconut in a large mixing bowl.

Place the remaining ingredients in a small saucepan over medium heat and stir until well combined and the chocolate has melted. Pour over the dried fruit and stir well to ensure the fruit is thoroughly coated in the chocolate mixture.

Place tablespoons of the chocolate fruit mixture on the baking tray and chill in the fridge for 2–3 hours or until firm.

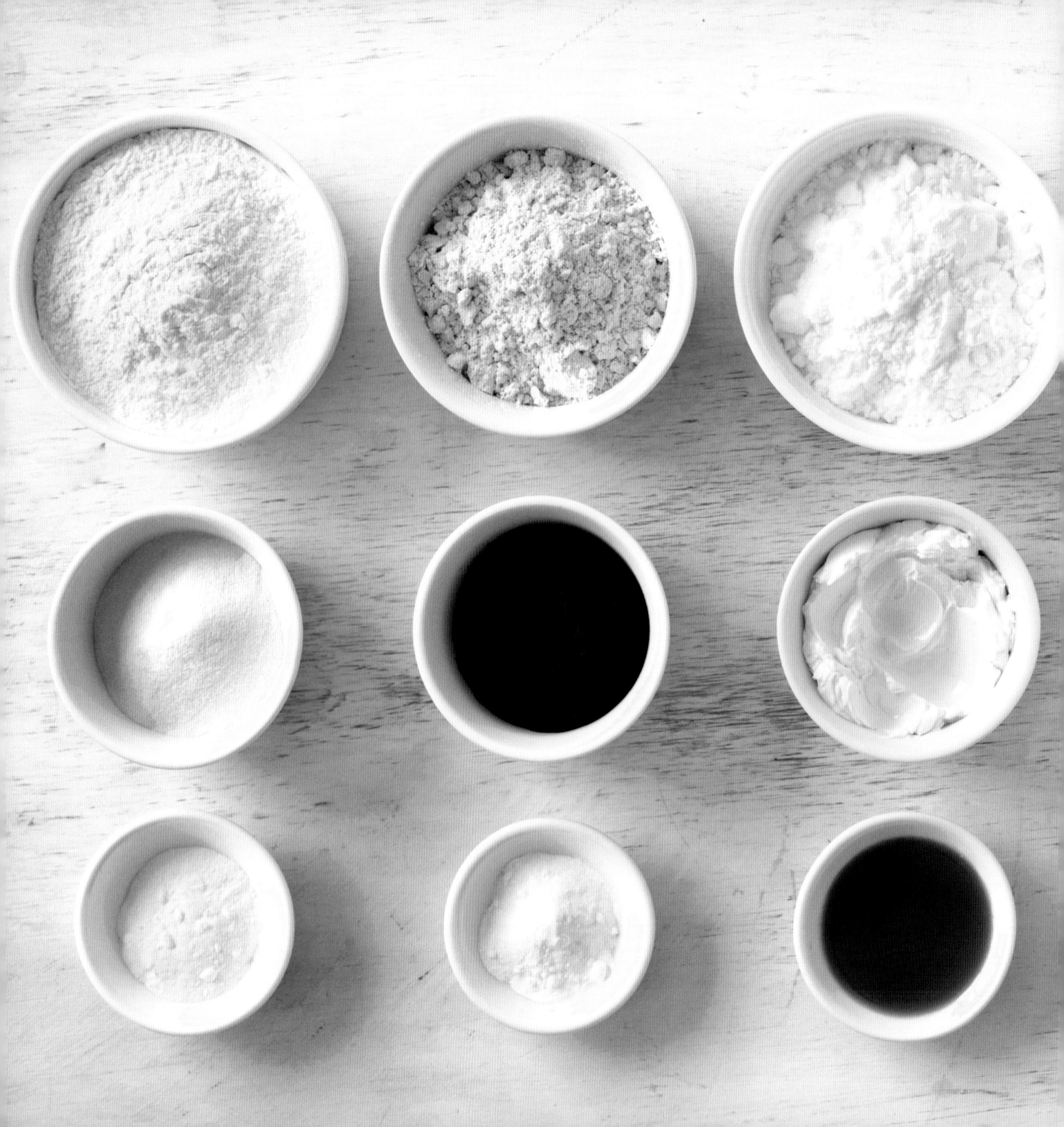

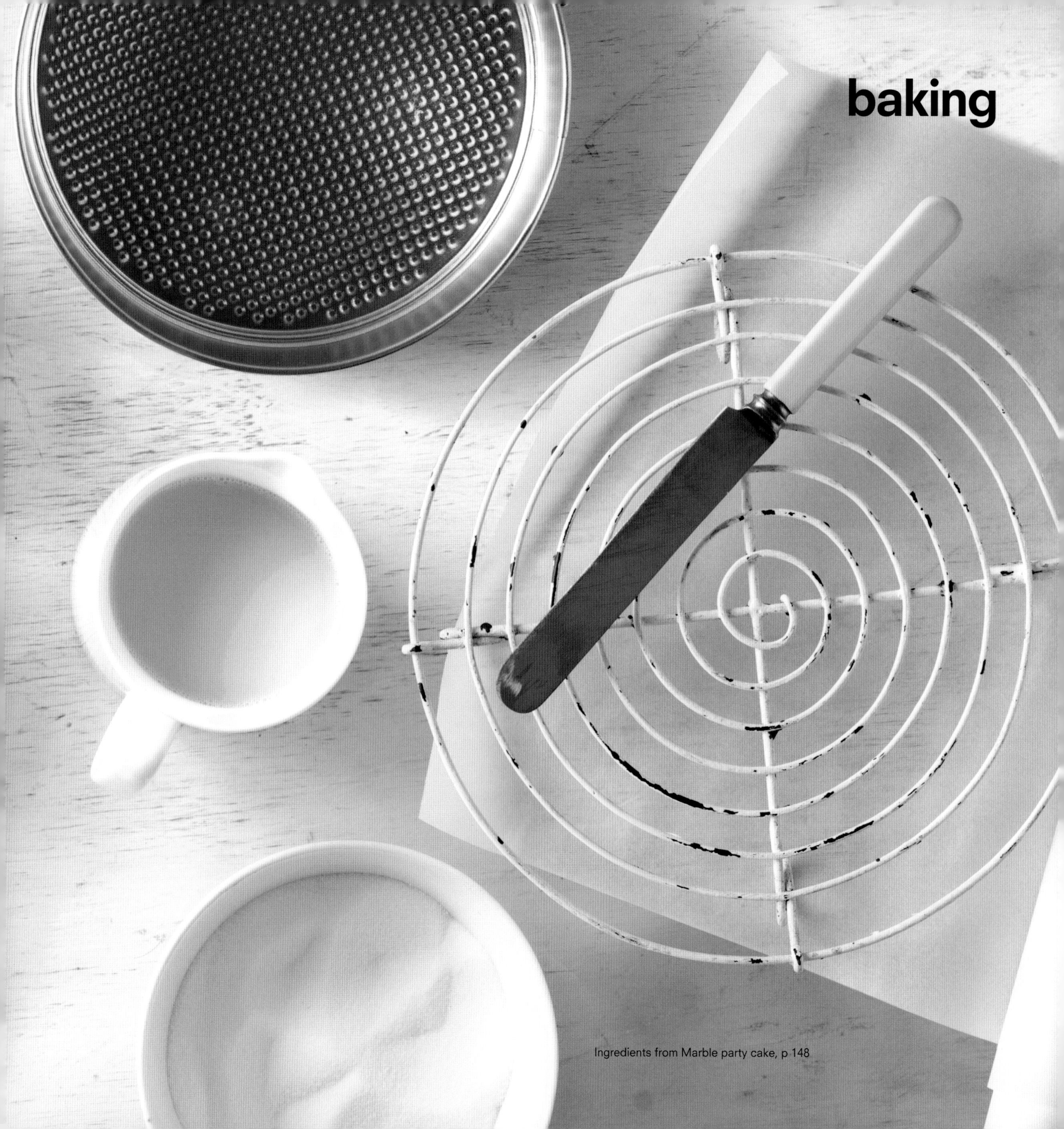

baking

Ingredients from Marble party cake, p 148

Marble party cake

Even if food allergies are an issue, a birthday cake isn't out of the question. This recipe shows how. You can make a vanilla-flavoured icing instead by omitting the cocoa and adding a splash of vanilla essence.

SERVES 10–12

2 cups (260 g) fine rice flour
1 cup (90 g) besan flour
1 cup (180 g) potato flour
1 tablespoon gluten-free baking powder
2 teaspoons bicarbonate of soda
2 teaspoons xanthan gum
120 g soy-free, dairy-free spread, melted
1 tablespoon vanilla essence
2 cups (500 ml) rice milk
4 eggs, lightly beaten*
2 cups (440 g) caster sugar
2 tablespoons cocoa powder
strawberries, to decorate (optional)

CHOCOLATE FROSTING
200 g soy-free, dairy-free spread
350 g pure icing sugar, sifted
75 g cocoa powder, sifted

Preheat the oven to 180°C and grease two 21 cm springform tins.

Sift the flours, baking powder, bicarbonate of soda and xanthan gum into a large bowl.

Place the melted spread, vanilla, rice milk, eggs and sugar in a large bowl and stir until well combined. Pour into the dry ingredients and stir with a large metal spoon for 2–3 minutes or until smooth.

Spoon half the batter into a separate bowl and sift in the cocoa powder. Mix with a wooden spoon until well combined. Divide the plain batter evenly between the two cake tins, then spoon the chocolate batter over the top. Use a flat-bladed knife to swirl the batter, creating a marbled effect.

Place the tins in the oven and bake for 30–35 minutes, then cover with foil and cook for further 30 minutes or until firm to the touch (a skewer inserted into the centre should come out clean). Rotate the tins halfway through the cooking time. Cool the cakes in the tins for 5 minutes, then turn out onto a large wire rack to cool completely.

To make the frosting, combine the spread, icing sugar, cocoa powder and 3 tablespoons water in a bowl and beat with hand-held electric beaters until smooth.

Spread about one third of the frosting over one cake, then place the second cake on top. Use the remaining frosting to ice the top and side of the sandwiched cake. Decorate with fresh strawberries (if using) and serve.

***For egg allergy**
Place 1¼ tablespoons psyllium husks in a small bowl and pour over 280 ml boiling water, stirring constantly to ensure the psyllium does not clump together. Set aside for 4–5 minutes until it forms a gel, stirring occasionally. Use in place of the egg.

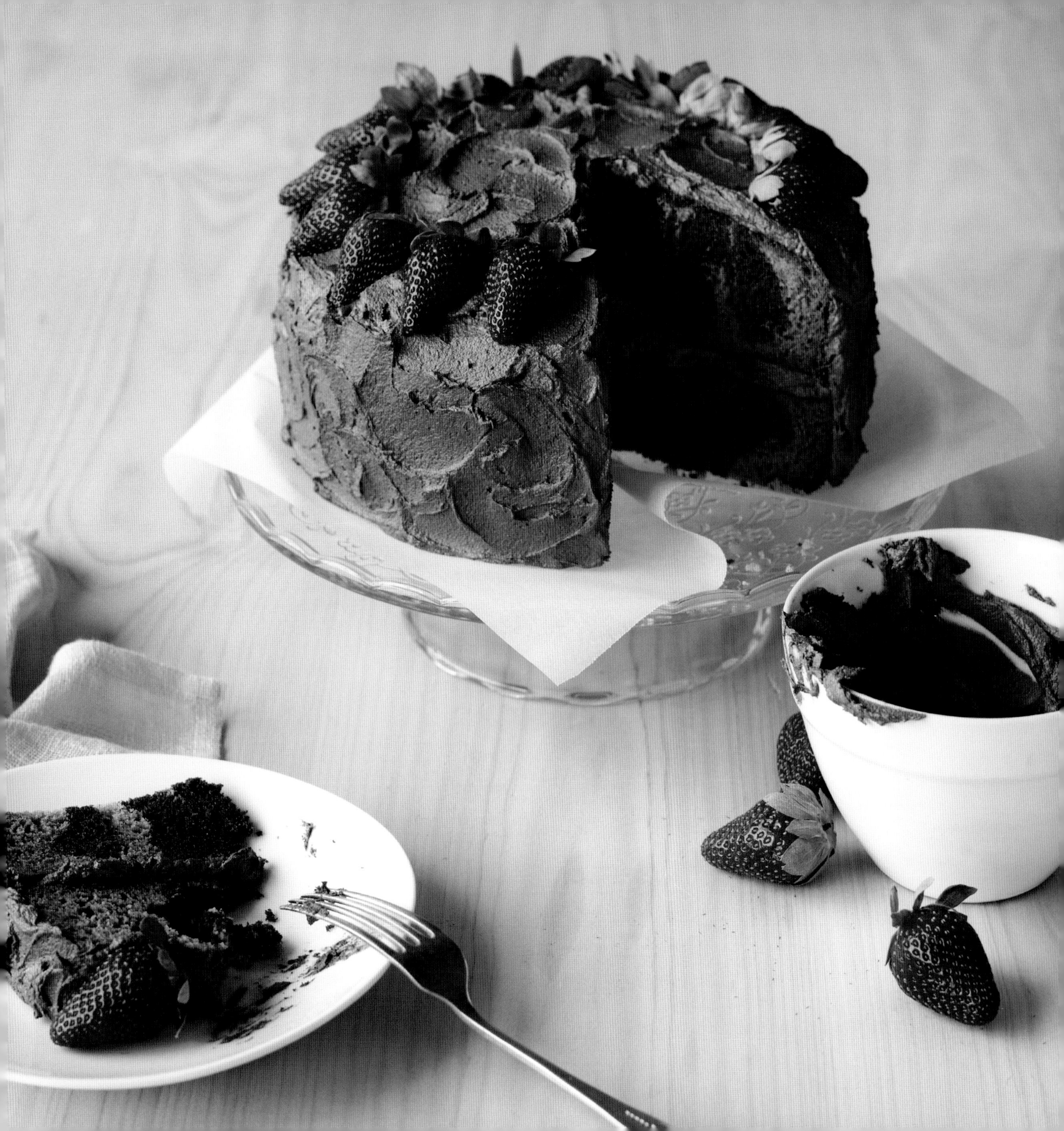

Apple and sultana rock cakes

The texture of rock cakes is softer than biscuits, but crisper than muffins. They can be made as tiny mouthfuls or larger mounds for a more substantial snack. In this version, the apple is enhanced with cinnamon. MAKES 16

3 tablespoons soy-free, dairy-free spread
3 tablespoons sugar
1 teaspoon vanilla essence
¾ cup (100 g) brown rice flour
½ cup (75 g) maize cornflour
½ teaspoon bicarbonate of soda
½ teaspoon xanthan gum
½ teaspoon mixed spice
¾ teaspoon ground cinnamon
1 egg, lightly beaten*
1 cup (60 g) roughly chopped dried apple
3 tablespoons sultanas

Preheat the oven to 170°C. Line a large baking tray with baking paper.

Place the spread, sugar and vanilla in a medium bowl and beat with a wooden spoon until creamy and well combined.

Sift the flours, bicarbonate of soda, xanthan gum, mixed spice and cinnamon into a large bowl. Add to the creamy spread mixture with the egg, dried apple, sultanas and 2 tablespoons warm water and fold in with a large metal spoon. Form the mixture into walnut-sized balls and place on the baking tray.

Bake for 12–15 minutes or until golden and firm to the touch. Allow to cool for 5 minutes on the tray, then transfer to a wire rack to cool completely.

***For egg allergy**

Place 1 teaspoon psyllium husks in a small bowl and pour over 3 tablespoons boiling water, stirring constantly to ensure the psyllium does not clump together. Set aside for 4–5 minutes until it forms a gel, stirring occasionally. Use in place of the egg.

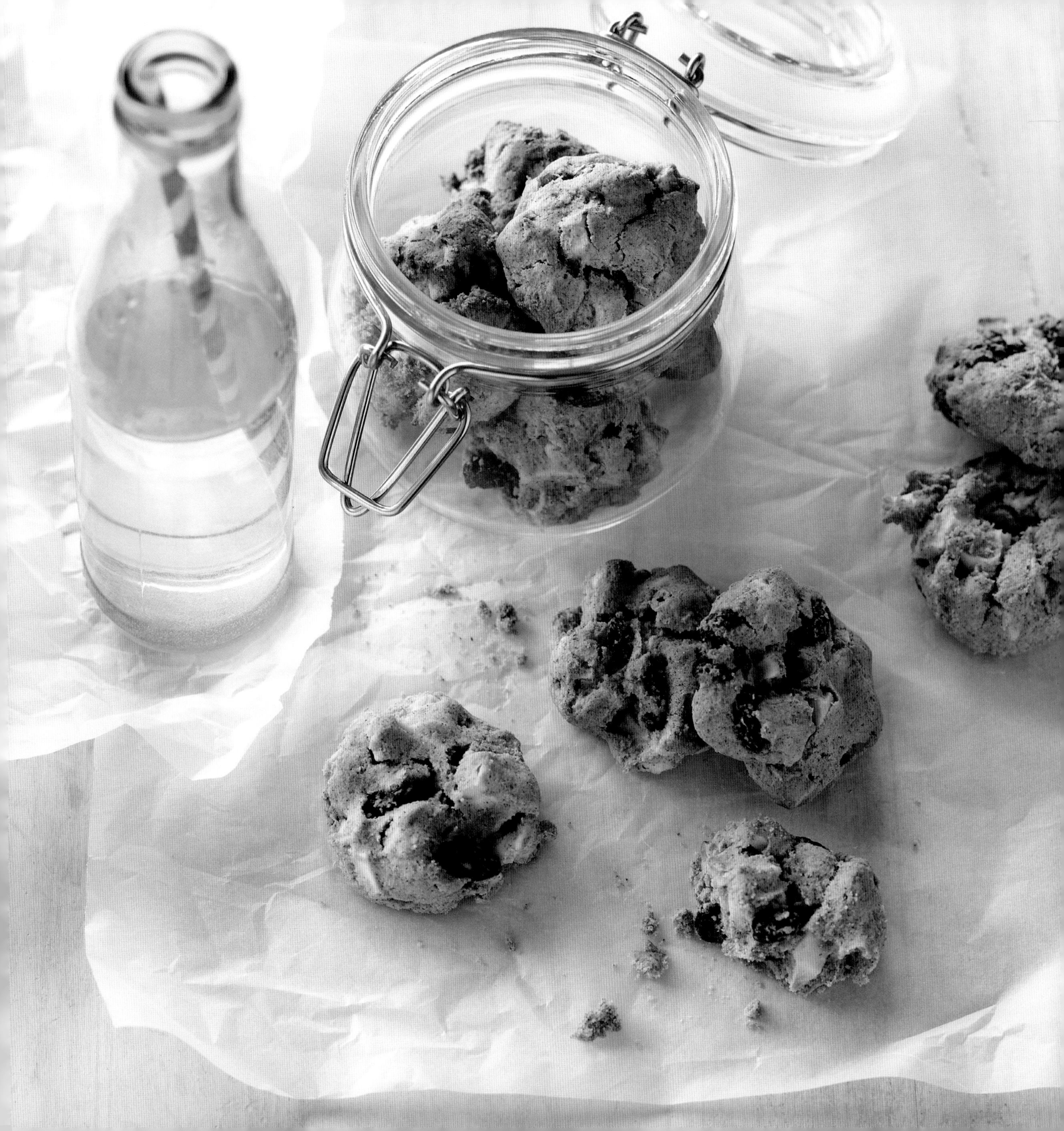

Date scones

Scones always make me think of happy times. These scones are flavoured with dates, so they don't really need a topping, however you may wish to serve them with jam. Make them with sultanas instead, if liked, or leave them plain.

MAKES 10

1 cup (150 g) maize cornflour
1 cup (125 g) tapioca flour
½ cup (45 g) besan flour
1 teaspoon xanthan gum
2 teaspoons gluten-free baking powder
3 tablespoons caster sugar
80 g soy-free, dairy-free spread, at room temperature, diced
1 egg*
150 ml rice milk
½ cup (70 g) roughly chopped pitted dates
soy-free, dairy-free spread and strawberry jam, to serve (optional)

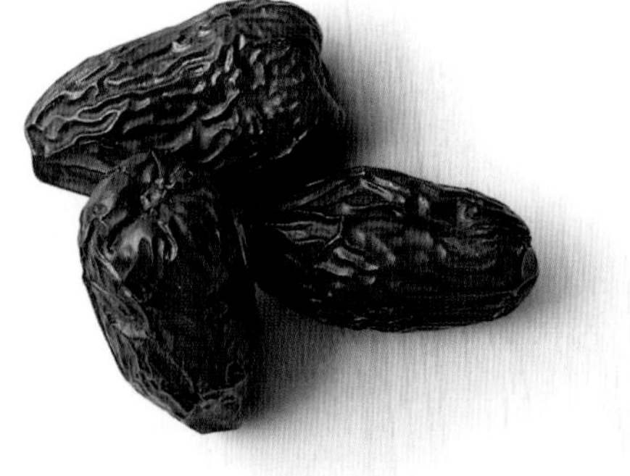

Preheat the oven to 200°C. Line a baking tray with baking paper.

Sift the flours, xanthan gum, baking powder and sugar into a medium bowl. Rub in the spread with your fingertips until the mixture resembles fine breadcrumbs. Add the egg, rice milk and dates all at once and mix with a large metal spoon until the mixture just begins to hold together.

Gently bring the dough together with your hands and let it rest in the bowl for 5 minutes. Turn it out onto a lightly floured surface and knead gently with your hands, pressing and turning it four or five times until the dough is smooth.

Using a lightly floured rolling pin, roll out the dough to a thickness of 2.5 cm and cut out 10 scones with a 5 cm round cutter. Use a straight-down motion to do this – if you twist the cutter, the scones will rise unevenly during cooking. It's a good idea to dip the cutter in cornflour before cutting out each scone to prevent sticking. Place the scones on the tray about 1 cm apart and bake for 10–12 minutes or until golden and cooked through.

Remove the scones from the oven and immediately wrap them in a clean tea towel (this will help give them a soft crust). Serve warm with spread and jam, if liked.

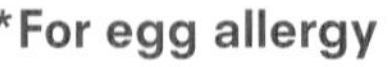

***For egg allergy**
Omit the egg and increase the rice milk to 200 ml.

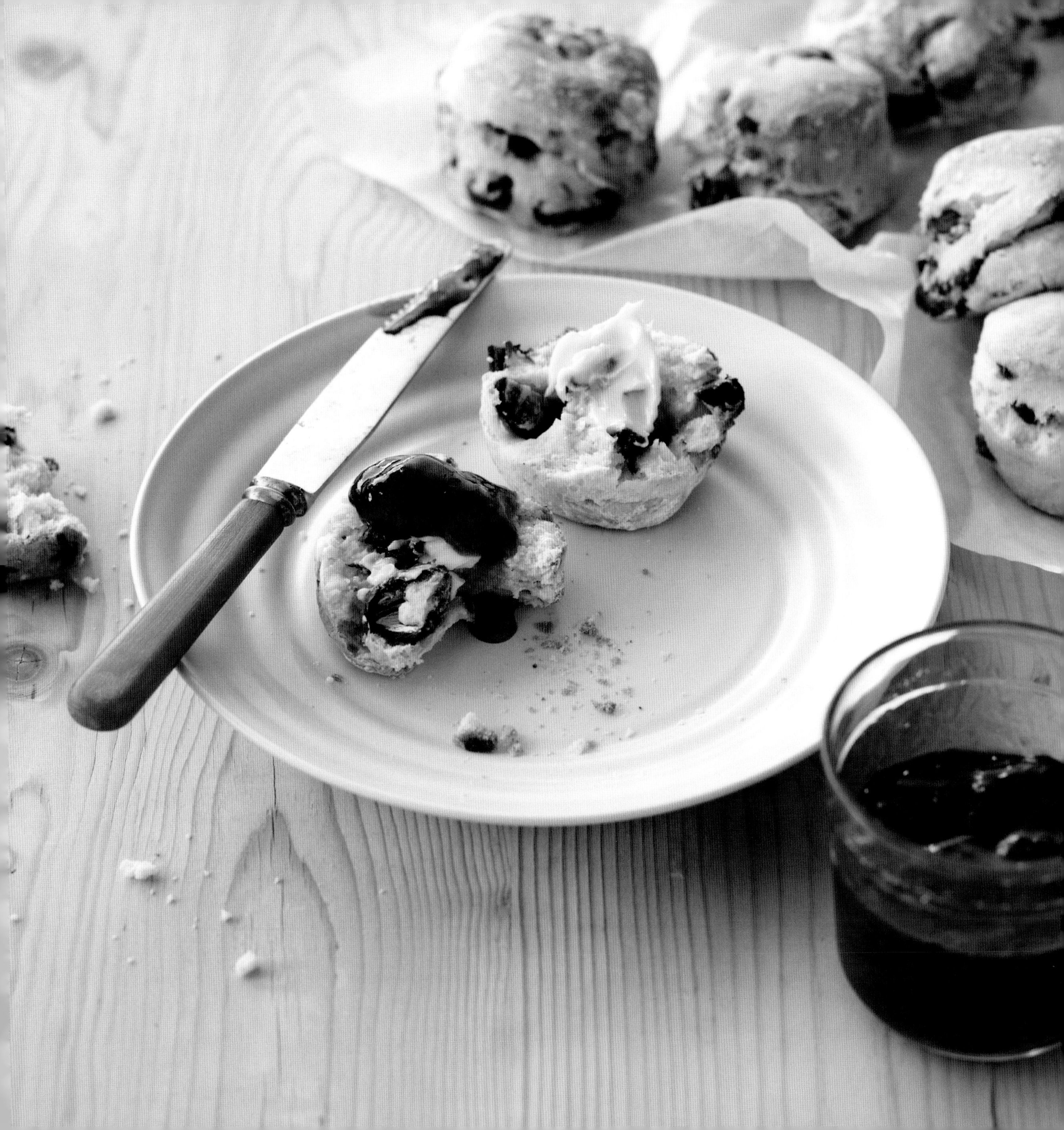

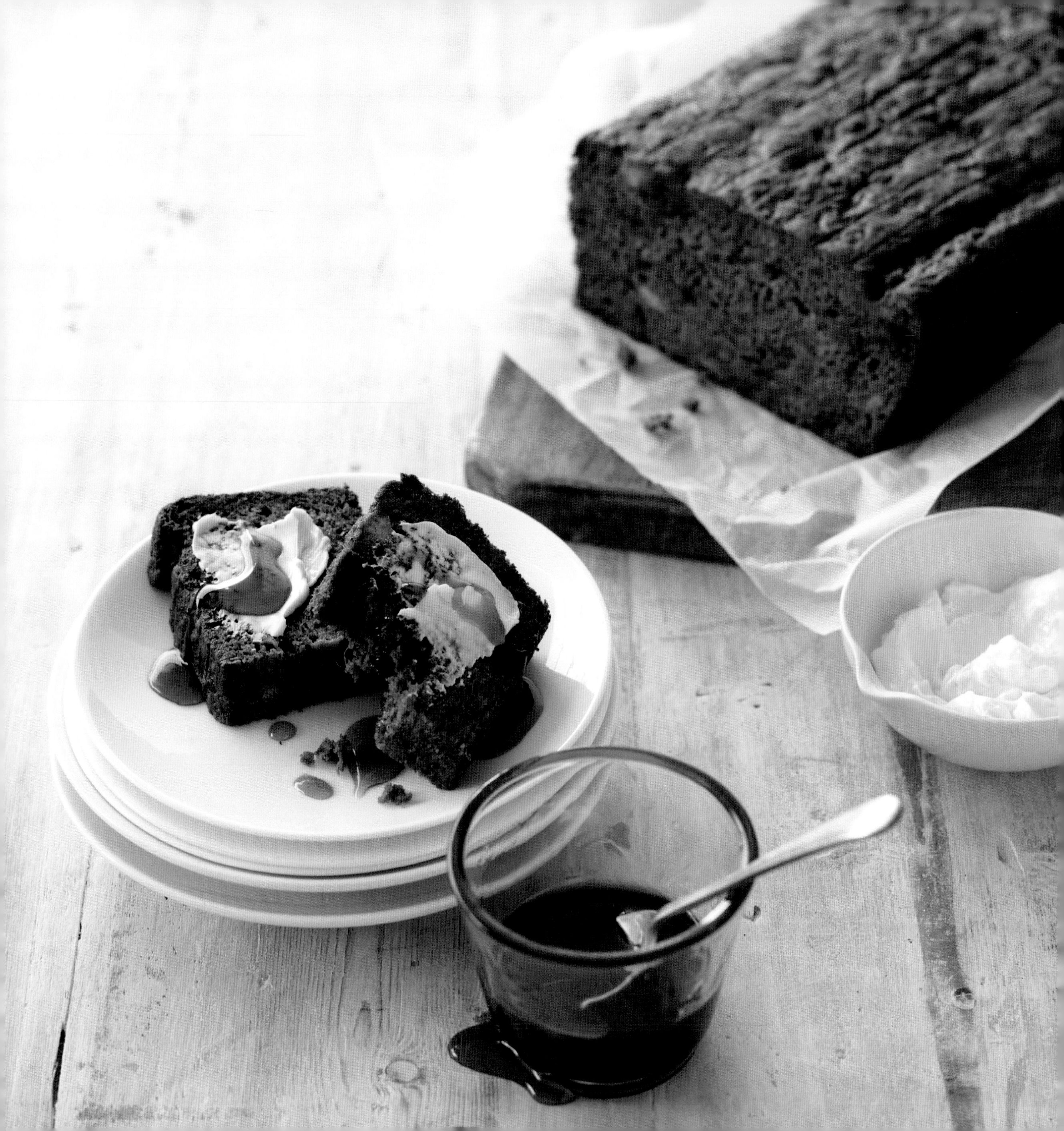

Banana and date loaf

Besan flour is made from chickpeas. It has similar baking properties to soy flour, so is a useful substitute if you are allergic to soy. It can be purchased in health-food shops and Indian groceries. SERVES 10

2 cups (280 g) coarsely chopped pitted dates
½ cup (110 g) brown sugar
1 cup (130 g) fine rice flour
3 tablespoons besan flour
3 tablespoons potato flour
2 teaspoons gluten-free baking powder
1 teaspoon bicarbonate of soda
1 teaspoon xanthan gum
2 teaspoons mixed spice
1 teaspoon ground cinnamon
2 ripe bananas
½ cup (125 ml) rice milk
2 eggs, lightly beaten*
soy-free, dairy-free spread and maple syrup, to serve (optional)

Place the dates, sugar and 1½ cups (375 ml) water in a large saucepan over medium–high heat and cook, stirring, until the sugar has dissolved and the water is almost boiling. Reduce the heat to medium–low and simmer for 10 minutes. Remove from the heat and allow to cool completely.

Preheat the oven to 170°C and grease a 23 cm × 13 cm × 7 cm loaf tin.

Sift the flours, baking powder, bicarbonate of soda, xanthan gum, mixed spice and cinnamon into a large mixing bowl.

Mash the bananas in a small bowl, then add the rice milk and mix together well. Add to the dry ingredients with the egg and cooled date mixture. Stir with a wooden spoon until well combined.

Spoon the batter into the tin and bake for 45 minutes, then cover with foil and cook for a further 15–20 minutes or until firm to the touch (a skewer should come out clean when inserted into the centre of cake). Cool in the tin for 5 minutes, then turn out onto a wire rack to cool completely. Serve with spread and maple syrup, if liked.

***For egg allergy**
Place 2½ teaspoons psyllium husks in a small bowl and pour over ½ cup (125 ml) boiling water, stirring constantly to ensure the psyllium does not clump together. Set aside for 4–5 minutes until it forms a gel, stirring occasionally. Use in place of the egg.

Cranberry and sultana muffins

Wheat-free baking requires a combination of flours, as there is no single flour that is a direct equivalent of wheat. The flours described here produce the right texture for muffins. MAKES 12

1 cup (170 g) brown rice flour
½ cup (75 g) maize cornflour
½ cup (90 g) potato flour
1 teaspoon bicarbonate of soda
2 teaspoons gluten-free baking powder
1 teaspoon xanthan gum
½ teaspoon mixed spice
1 teaspoon ground cinnamon
2 tablespoons soy-free, dairy-free spread, melted
1½ cups (375 ml) rice milk
1 egg, lightly beaten*
½ cup (80 g) sultanas
½ cup (65 g) dried cranberries (craisins)
1 cup (220 g) caster sugar

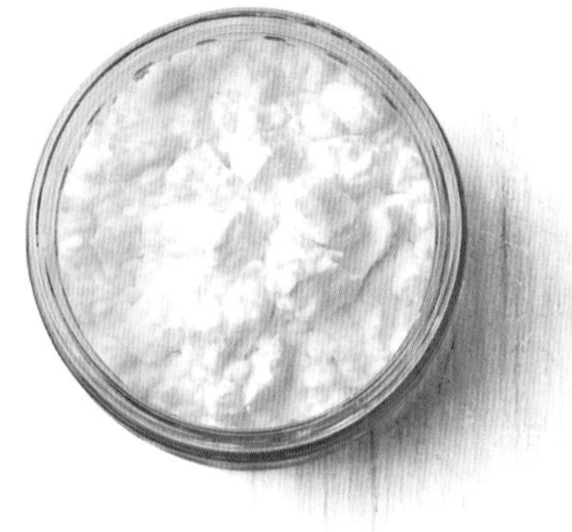

Preheat the oven to 170°C. Grease a 12-hole muffin tin or line with paper cases.

Sift the flours, bicarbonate of soda, baking powder, xanthan gum, mixed spice and cinnamon into a large mixing bowl.

Combine the melted spread, rice milk and egg in a medium bowl. Stir in the sultanas, cranberries and sugar, then add to the dry ingredients and mix with a wooden spoon until combined.

Spoon the batter into the muffin holes and cook for 12–15 minutes or until golden and a skewer comes out clean when inserted into the centre of the muffin. Cool in the tin for 5 minutes, then transfer to a wire rack to cool completely.

***For egg allergy**
Place 1 teaspoon psyllium husks in a small bowl and pour over 3 tablespoons boiling water, stirring constantly to ensure the psyllium does not clump together. Set aside for 4–5 minutes until it forms a gel, stirring occasionally. Use in place of the egg.

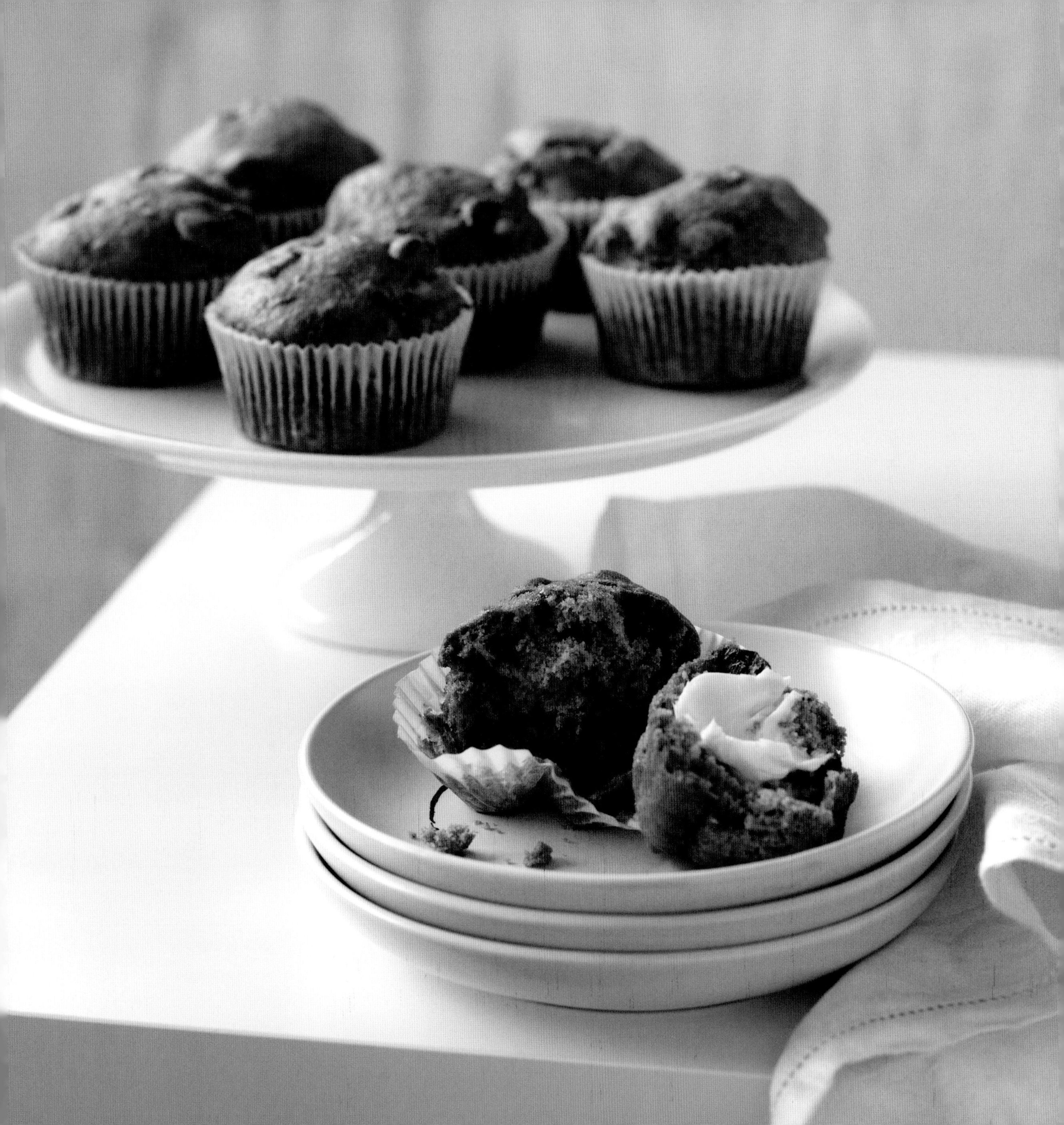

Ginger marmalade biscuits

Depending on what you have in your pantry, you can replace the rice, maize and besan flours with an equal quantity of commercial gluten-free, wheat-free plain flour, if liked. Just make sure you check it's soy-free if you're allergic to soy.

MAKES ABOUT 20

125 g soy-free, dairy-free spread
1 teaspoon vanilla essence
3 tablespoons brown sugar
3 tablespoons caster sugar
⅔ cup (85 g) fine rice flour
½ cup (75 g) maize cornflour
3 tablespoons besan flour
½ teaspoon bicarbonate of soda
1 teaspoon xanthan gum
2 teaspoons ground ginger
1 egg, lightly beaten*
2 tablespoons orange marmalade
60 g crystallised ginger, roughly chopped

Preheat the oven to 170°C. Grease two baking trays or line with baking paper.

Place the spread, vanilla and sugars in a medium bowl and beat with hand-held electric beaters until the mixture is creamy and well combined.

Sift the flours, bicarbonate of soda, xanthan gum and ground ginger into a large bowl. Add the creamy spread mixture and egg and beat well with a wooden spoon. Stir in the marmalade and crystallised ginger.

Place tablespoons of the mixture onto the trays, leaving room for spreading. Bake for 8–10 minutes or until lightly golden. Cool on the trays for 5 minutes, then transfer to a wire rack to cool completely.

***For egg allergy**
Place 1 teaspoon psyllium husks in a small bowl and pour over 3 tablespoons boiling water, stirring constantly to ensure the psyllium does not clump together. Set aside for 4–5 minutes until it forms a gel, stirring occasionally. Use in place of the egg.

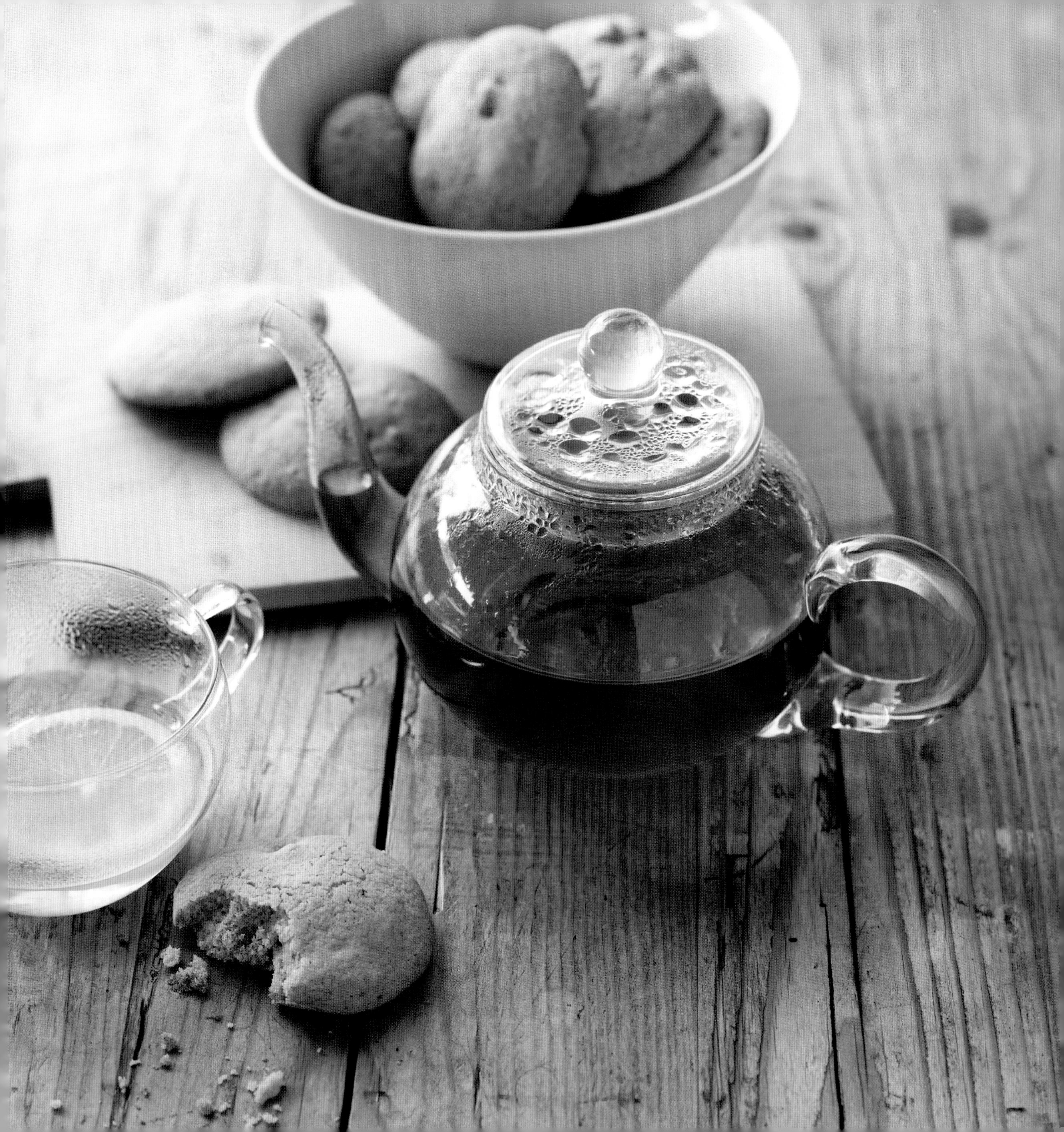

Chocolate cake

This is an everyday chocolate cake that is great for school lunchboxes, or it can be dressed up for dessert. I've used vanilla frosting here but you could also use a chocolate icing, if preferred (see page 148). SERVES 10

1 cup (130 g) fine rice flour
½ cup (45 g) besan flour
½ cup (90 g) potato flour
⅔ cup (70 g) cocoa powder
1 teaspoon bicarbonate of soda
2 teaspoons gluten-free baking powder
1 teaspoon xanthan gum
3 tablespoons soy-free, dairy-free spread, melted
2 teaspoons vanilla essence
1 cup (250 ml) rice milk
2 eggs, lightly beaten*
1½ cups (330 g) caster sugar

VANILLA FROSTING
200 g gluten-free, wheat-free, dairy-free, soy-free, nut-free white chocolate
85 g dairy-free, soy-free spread
50 g pure icing sugar
1–2 tablespoons boiling water

Preheat the oven to 180°C and grease a 19 cm springform cake tin.

Sift the flours, cocoa powder, bicarbonate of soda, baking powder and xanthan gum into a large bowl.

Place the spread, vanilla, rice milk, egg and sugar in a medium bowl and mix together well. Add to the dry ingredients and beat with hand-held electric beaters for 2–3 minutes.

Pour the batter into the tin and bake for 35–40 minutes. Cover with foil and cook for a further 10–15 minutes or until firm to the touch (a skewer inserted into the centre should come out clean). Cool in the tin for 5 minutes, then turn out onto a wire rack to cool completely.

To make the frosting, place the chocolate and spread in a medium glass bowl. Set over a saucepan of simmering water (make sure the base of the bowl does not touch the water) and stir until melted and combined. Take the bowl off the heat and stir in the icing sugar. Gradually stir in enough boiling water to achieve a spreadable consistency. Spread over the cooled cake.

***For egg allergy**
Place 2½ teaspoons psyllium husks in a small bowl and pour over 140 ml boiling water, stirring constantly to ensure the psyllium does not clump together. Set aside for 4–5 minutes until it forms a gel, stirring occasionally. Use in place of the egg.

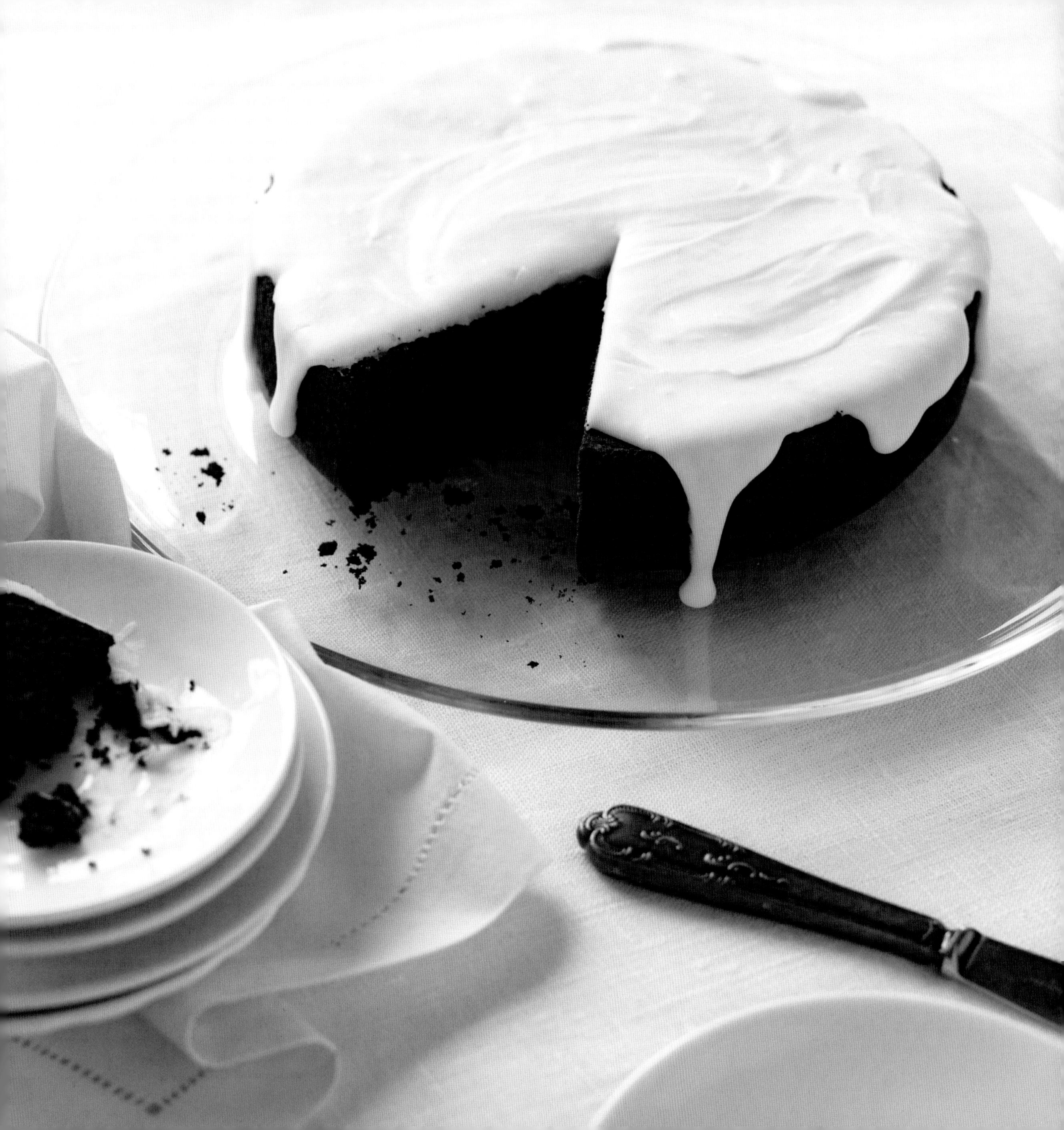

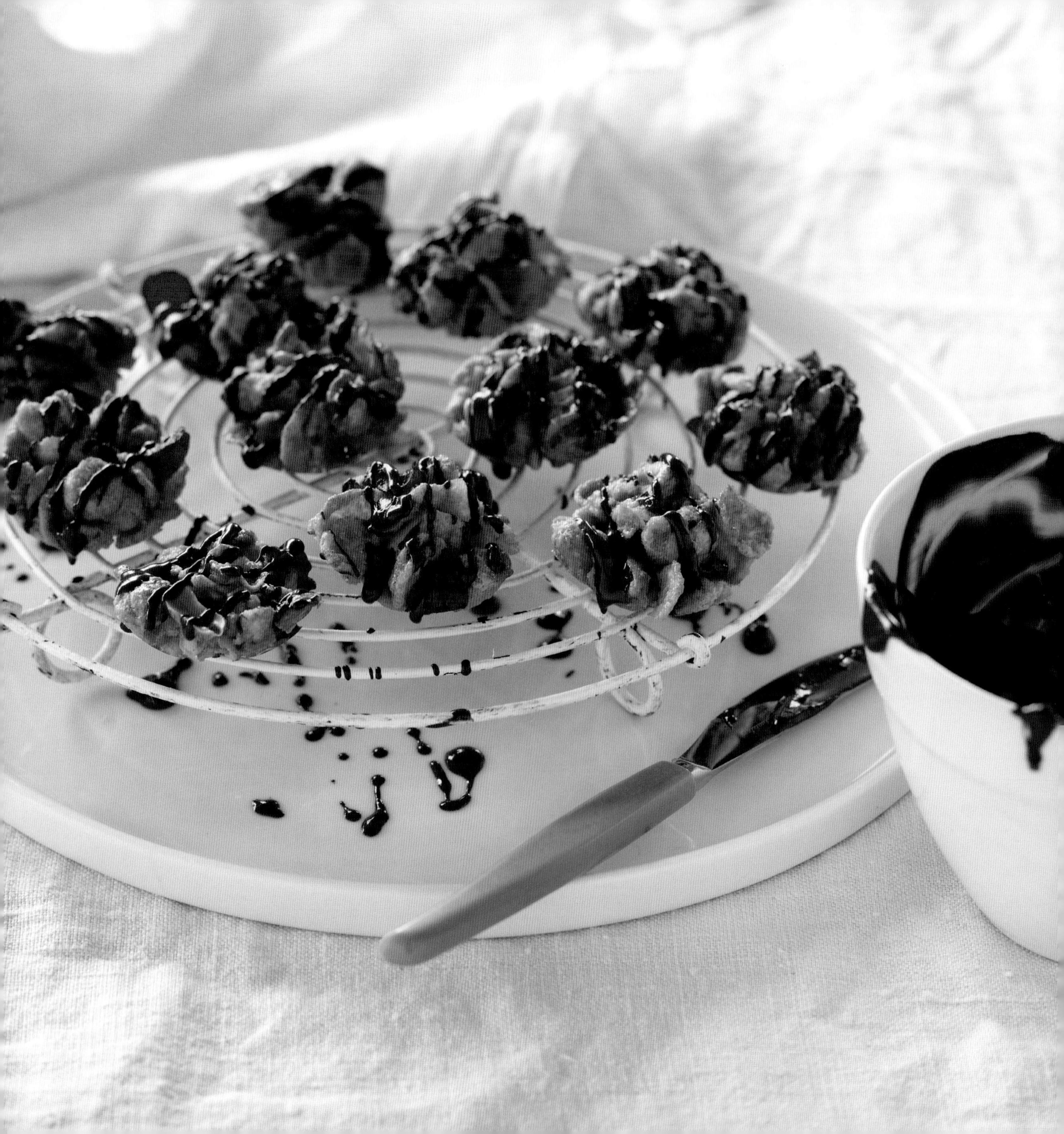

Florentine bundles

Florentine biscuits often have nuts in them, but not this scrumptious variation. If you're not allergic to peanuts, you could add 3–4 tablespoons of roughly chopped unsalted peanuts with the glace cherries, if you wish.

MAKES 24

½ cup (110 g) caster sugar
3 tablespoons brown sugar
75 g soy-free, dairy-free spread
2 tablespoons rice milk
3 cups (120 g) gluten-free, wheat-free cornflakes
½ cup (100 g) roughly chopped glace cherries
100 g gluten-free, wheat-free, dairy-free, soy-free, nut-free dark chocolate

Preheat the oven to 175°C. Line two 12-hole patty pan tins with paper cases.

Place the sugars, spread and rice milk in a small saucepan over low heat and stir until the sugar has dissolved and the spread has melted. Simmer gently for 5–8 minutes or until the mixture has browned and thickened. Remove from the heat and set aside to cool for 5 minutes.

Combine the cornflakes and glace cherries in a medium mixing bowl, add the sugar mixture and stir well with a wooden spoon.

Spoon 2 tablespoons of the mixture into each paper case. Don't worry if the mixture doesn't seem to be holding together – it will when it's cooked.

Bake for 6–8 minutes or until golden. If they have spread too thin during baking, use a flat-bladed knife to carefully push the hot toffee back towards the centre of the biscuit. Cool in the tin for 15 minutes then transfer to a large wire rack to cool completely.

Place the chocolate in a small glass bowl set over a saucepan of simmering water (make sure the base of the bowl does not touch the water) and stir until melted. Drizzle the chocolate over the cooled biscuits and leave to set at room temperature.

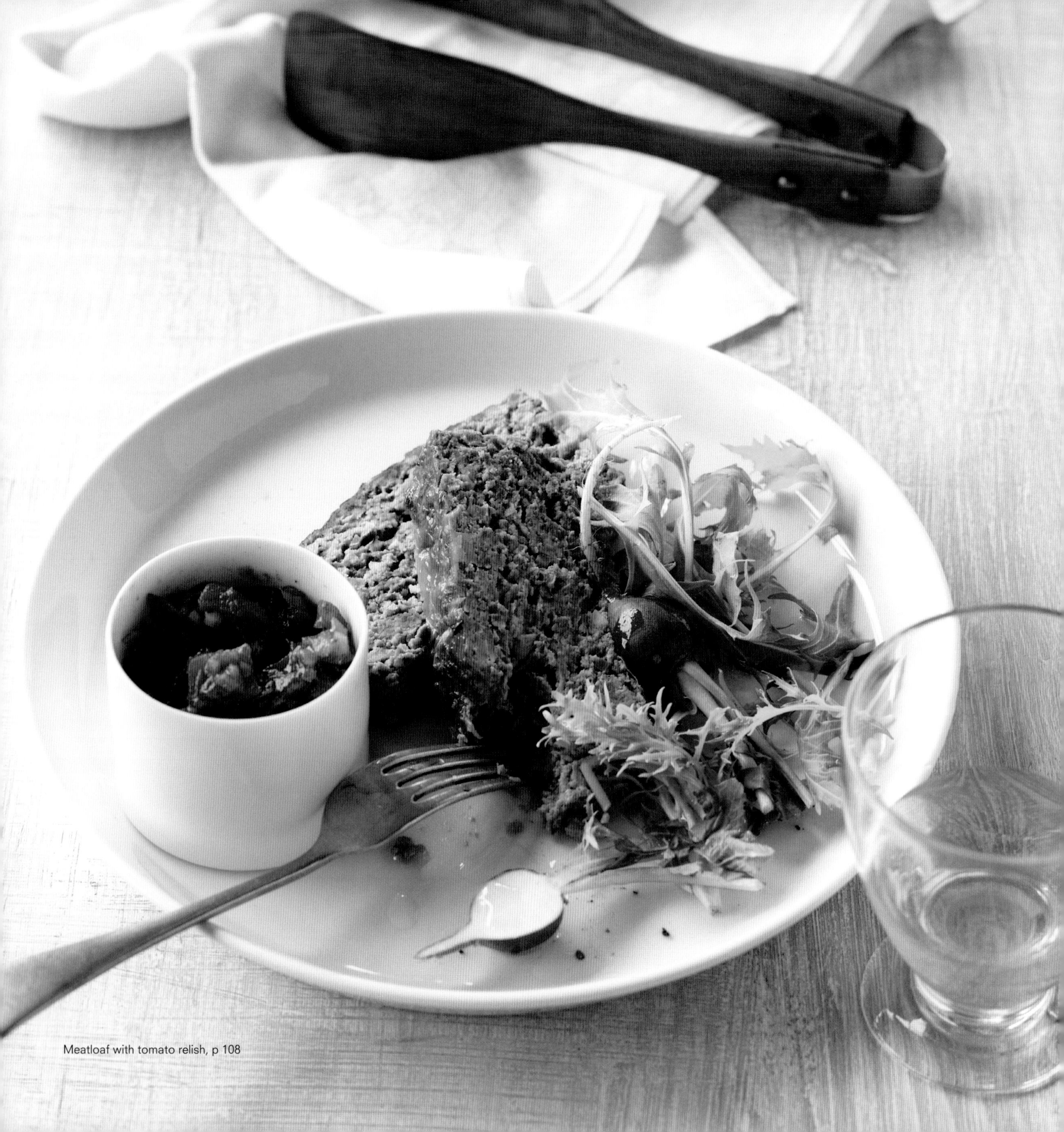

Meatloaf with tomato relish, p 108

acknowledgements

I would like to extend heartfelt thanks to the fantastic team at Penguin for inviting me to write this collection of recipes for people with food allergies. You have prioritised the needs of people with special dietary requirements, and enthusiastically supported me in my goal to promote enjoyment of food.

I have thoroughly enjoyed the strong and rewarding working relationship that I have with you all. Thank you Julie Gibbs: it is a privilege to work with you again. I would especially like to thank Rachel Carter, the most magnificent editor one could hope for; Rob Palmer, who is one of the most amazing food photographers and always takes the most gorgeous photos of my recipes; stylist Michelle Noerianto and home economist Lucy Busuttil who made the food look so delicious; and Ricardo Felipe for his stunning layout and design. Thank you so much – together we have produced a book we can be immensely proud of.

To my beautiful family – Mum, Dad, Linda, Gra, Zoe, Joel, Em, Mark, Ang, Nana S, Nana B, Sarah and Marc – thank you. You are enormously important to me and so loved. I thank you for the strength, encouragement, love and support you give me. And of course to my close special friends: you are all so dear to me.

To the friends, colleagues and acquaintances I have not specifically mentioned, I thank you for your very special role in helping to make my life so fulfilling.

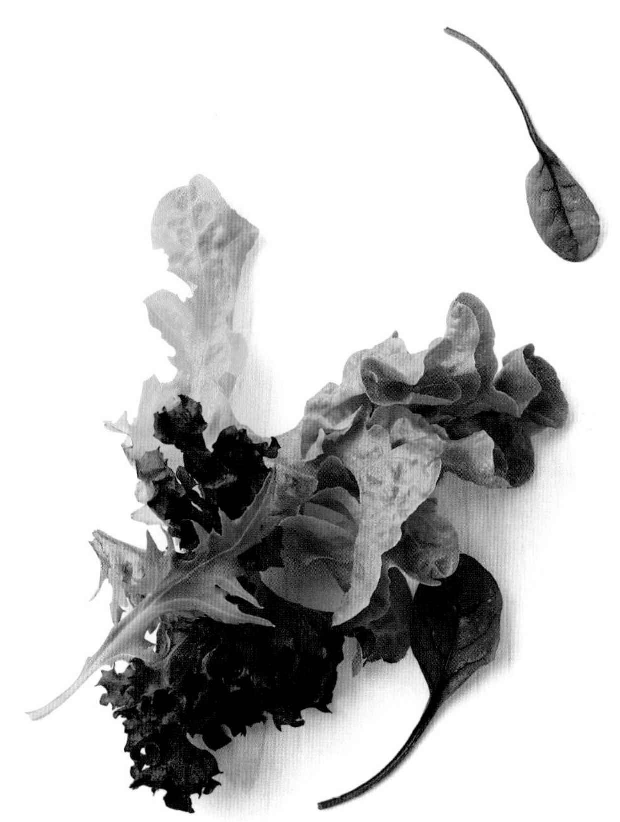

index

additives containing
  allergens 10

allergens 2
  common foods
    containing 8–11
  on food labels 4–5
  identifying 4

allergies
  body's reaction to 2
  in children 3, 4
  diagnosing 3
  'food traps' 7, 8–10
  how long do they last? 3, 4
  prevalence 3
  symptoms 2, 3
  testing for 2, 3–4
  treating 4
  what are they? 2

allergy-free foods
  recipes 11
  stocking your kitchen 6–7
  where to buy 6, 7

amaranth flour 6

anaphylaxis 2, 5

apples
  Apple and sultana
    rock cakes 150
  Jamaican apple tart 136
  Rhubarb, raspberry and
    apple crumble 129

arrowroot flour 6

Asian chicken coleslaw 20

Asparagus and corn bites 83

Australasian Society of Clinical
  Immunology and Allergy 4

avocados
  Choc-orange mousse 134
  Garden salad
    with avocado 22

bacon
  Bacon and tomato
    stuffed mushrooms 15
  Baked potatoes with chilli
    beef and bacon 68

Baked beef rendang risotto 59

baked goods 9

Baked potatoes with chilli beef
  and bacon 68

bananas
  Banana breakfast
    smoothie 14
  Banana and date loaf 155
  Self-saucing banana pudding
    with caramel sauce 140

barley products 5

battered foods 10

beans, green
  Sweet potato, prosciutto
    and green bean salad 26

beans, tinned
  Beef burritos 111
  Chilli con carne 56

beef
  Baked beef rendang
    risotto 59
  Baked potatoes with
    chilli beef and bacon 68
  Beef burritos 111
  Beef with herb 'butter' 52
  Beef in plum sauce 70
  Chilli con carne 56
  Creole beef with
    crispy potatoes 60
  Kofta balls 83
  Meatloaf with
    tomato relish 108
  Porcupine meatballs 106
  Spring rolls 82

berries
  Cherry berry jelly cups 124
  Rhubarb, raspberry and
    apple crumble 129

besan flour 6, 155

Bircher muesli 15

biscuits
  Florentine bundles 163
  Ginger marmalade
    biscuits 158

breads, allergens in 8

brown rice flour 6

buckwheat flour 6
  Buckwheat crepes
    with chicken and
    tarragon filling 39

burritos
  Beef burritos 111

cabbage
  Asian chicken coleslaw 20
  Chow mein 76
  Spring rolls 82

cakes
  Apple and sultana
    rock cakes 150
  Chocolate cake 160
  Marble party cake 148

capsicum
  Curried spinach and
    capsicum kasha 98
  Ratatouille 90
  Roast capsicum and
    tomato sauce 88
  Spinach and capsicum
    muffins 14

caramel
  Caramel popcorn 124
  Caramel sauce 132, 140
  Chilli caramel sauce 42

casserole
  Curried sausage
    casserole 112

cereals, allergens in 8

Chargrilled chicken with mango
  and cucumber salsa 32

Cherry berry jelly cups 124

chicken
  Asian chicken coleslaw 20
  Buckwheat crepes
    with chicken and
    tarragon filling 39
  Chargrilled chicken with
    mango and cucumber
    salsa 32
  Chicken with chilli
    caramel sauce 42
  Chicken and corn soup 40
  Chicken fried rice 104
  Chicken pilaf 34
  Chicken with sage
    'butter' sauce 42
  Lemon pepper
    chicken legs 116
  Mediterranean chicken
    pockets 45
  Quick Thai chicken risotto 46
  Smoked chicken pasta 36

chickpeas
  Chickpea salad with
    zucchini and chilli 18
  Chickpeas with ratatouille 90
  Falafels 87

chilli
  Baked potatoes with
    chilli beef and bacon 68
  Chickpea salad with
    zucchini and chilli 18
  Chilli caramel sauce 42
  Chilli con carne 56

chocolate
  Choc-honey clusters
    with dried fruit 145
  Chocolate cake 160
  Chocolate frosting 148
  Choc-orange mousse 134
  Chocolate pancakes
    with caramel sauce 132
  Fruit kebabs with chocolate
    dipping sauce 125
  Rocky road 145

Chow mein 76

Chunky tomato and
  olive sauce 62

Citrus fennel salad 18

Citrus glaze 78

coconut
  Coconut rice pudding 142
  Rocky road 145

coeliac disease 3

compound ingredients 5

condiments, allergens in 10

confectionery, allergens in 9

cooking methods,
  allergens in 10

corn
  Asparagus and corn
    bites 83
  Chicken and corn soup 40
  Corn fritters with fresh
    tomato salsa 115

cornflour 6

Cranberry and
  sultana muffins 156

Creole beef with
  crispy potatoes 60

crepes
  Buckwheat crepes
    with chicken and
    tarragon filling 39

crumbles
  Rhubarb, raspberry and
    apple crumble 129

cucumber
  Mango and
    cucumber salsa 32

cuisines, allergens in 9

Curried sausage
  casserole 112

Curried spinach and
  capsicum kasha 98

custard
  Custard topping 124
  Fruit custard flan 139

dairy and dairy-equivalent
  products 8

dates
  Banana and date loaf 155
  Date scones 152

desserts, allergens in 9

dried fruit
  Apple and sultana
    rock cakes 150
  Choc-honey clusters
    with dried fruit 145
  Cranberry and
    sultana muffins 156
  see also dates

drinks
  allergens in 10
  Banana breakfast smoothie 14
  Fruit punch 124

eggs and egg products 2, 4, 5, 8

eggplant
  Ratatouille 90
  Roast eggplant pilaf with
    Middle Eastern spices 101

elimination diet 2, 3–4

Falafels 87

false positive test results 3

fats and oils
  containing allergens 8

fennel
  Citrus fennel salad 18

Fig and prosciutto salad
  with spiced quail 28

fish and fish
  products 2, 3, 4, 5, 8

flans
  Fruit custard flan 139

Florentine bundles 163

flour alternatives to wheat
  and soy 6

FODMAPS 3

food additives, allergens in 10

food allergies *see* allergies

food hypersensitivity 2–3

food intolerance 2

food labels 4–5

Fresh tomato salsa 115

fried food
  Chicken fried rice 104
  containing allergens 10
  Fried brown rice 59

fritters
  Corn fritters with fresh
    tomato salsa 115

frosting
  Chocolate frosting 148
  Vanilla frosting 160

fruit
  allergens in 8
  Fruit custard flan 139
  Fruit kebabs with chocolate
    dipping sauce 125
  Fruit punch 124
  Citrus fennel salad 18

Garden salad with avocado 22

Garlic and herb gnocchi
  with roast capsicum and
  tomato sauce 88

Garlic pepper lamb stir-fry 72

Garlic and rosemary polenta 64

Ginger marmalade biscuits 158

gluten 2

gluten-containing grains 5

gluten-free flour 6

Gluten-free, wheat-free,
  dairy-free, egg-free, nut-free,
  soy-free pastry 136

gnocchi
  Garlic and herb gnocchi
    with roast capsicum and
    tomato sauce 88

ham
  Pea and ham soup 67

Hearty vegetable soup 94

herbs
  Buckwheat crepes
    with chicken and
    tarragon filling 39
  Garlic and herb gnocchi
    with roast capsicum and
    tomato sauce 88
  Garlic and rosemary
    polenta 64
  Herb 'butter' 52
    Herb-crusted rack of lamb
    with minted pea puree 51
  Herbed wedges 116
  Minted pea puree 51
  Quinoa salad with mint
    and lemon 25
  Sage 'butter' sauce 42
  Spinach, pumpkin and
    sage polenta slice 92

histamine 2

honey
  Choc-honey clusters
    with dried fruit 145

irritable bowel syndrome 3

Jamaican apple tart 136

jelly
  Cherry berry jelly cups 124

kasha
  Curried spinach and
    capsicum kasha 98

kids, meals for
  Beef burritos 111
  Chicken fried rice 104
  Corn fritters with fresh
    tomato salsa 115
  Curried sausage casserole 112
  Herbed wedges 116
  Lamb and vegetable stew 121
  Lemon pepper
    chicken legs 116
  Meatloaf with
    tomato relish 108
  Porcupine meatballs 106
  Pork spare ribs 118

kids, sweets for
  Caramel popcorn 124
  Cherry berry jelly cups 124
  Custard topping 124
  Fruit kebabs with chocolate
    dipping sauce 125
  Fruit punch 124

Kofta balls 83

lamb
- Garlic pepper lamb stir-fry 72
- Herb-crusted rack of lamb with minted pea puree 51
- Lamb shank and vegetable soup 54
- Lamb shanks with garlic and rosemary polenta 64
- Lamb and vegetable stew 121

lemons
- Lemon pepper chicken legs 116
- Quinoa salad with mint and lemon 25

Lentil soup 94

loaves
- Banana and date loaf 155

Mango and cucumber salsa 32

Marble party cake 148

marshmallows
- Rocky road 145

meat
- allergens in 8
- *see also* beef; lamb; pork; veal

meatballs
- Kofta balls 83
- Porcupine meatballs 106

Meatloaf with tomato relish 108

Mediterranean chicken pockets 45

milk and milk products 2, 4, 5

millet flour 6

Minted pea puree 51

mixed meals, allergens in 9

mousse
- Choc-orange mousse 134

muesli
- Bircher muesli 15

muffins
- Cranberry and sultana muffins 156
- Spinach and capsicum muffins 14

mushrooms
- Bacon and tomato stuffed mushrooms 15

oat products 5

olives
- Chunky tomato and olive sauce 62

oranges
- Citrus glaze 78
- Ginger marmalade biscuits 158

Osso buco 74

pancakes
- Chocolate pancakes with caramel sauce 132

Passionfruit puddings 130

pasta
- Smoked chicken pasta 36

pastry
- Gluten-free, wheat-free, dairy-free, egg-free, nut-free, soy-free pastry 136

peanuts and their products 2, 3, 4, 5

Pear and rocket salad 22

peas, dried
- Pea and ham soup 67

peas, green
- Minted pea puree 51

pilaf
- Chicken pilaf 34
- Roast eggplant pilaf with Middle Eastern spices 101

Plum sauce 70

polenta
- Garlic and rosemary polenta 64
- Spinach, pumpkin and sage polenta slice 92

popcorn
- Caramel popcorn 124

Porcupine meatballs 106

pork
- Chow mein 76
- Pork spare ribs 118
- Roast pork cutlets with citrus glaze 78
- San choi bow 82
- Spring rolls 82

potato flour 6

potatoes
- Baked potatoes with chilli beef and bacon 68
- Crispy potatoes 60
- Herbed wedges 116

prosciutto
- Fig and prosciutto salad with spiced quail 28
- Sweet potato, prosciutto and green bean salad 26

puddings
- Coconut rice pudding 142
- Passionfruit puddings 130
- Self-saucing banana pudding with caramel sauce 140

pumpkin
- Spinach, pumpkin and sage polenta slice 92
- Thai pumpkin soup 96

quail
- Fig and prosciutto salad with spiced quail 28

Quick Thai chicken risotto 46

quinoa flour 6

Quinoa salad with mint and lemon 25

RAST test 3

Ratatouille 90

relish
- Tomato relish 108

Rhubarb, raspberry and apple crumble 129

rice
- Asparagus and corn bites 83
- Chicken fried rice 104
- Coconut rice pudding 142
- Fried brown rice 59
- Mediterranean chicken pockets 45
- Porcupine meatballs 106
- *see also* pilaf; risotto

rice flour 6

risotto
- Baked beef rendang risotto 59
- Quick Thai chicken risotto 46

Roast capsicum and tomato sauce 88

Roast eggplant pilaf with Middle Eastern spices 101

Roast pork cutlets with citrus glaze 78

rock cakes
- Apple and sultana rock cakes 150

rocket
- Pear and rocket salad 22

Rocky road 145

royal jelly 5

rye products 5

salads
- Asian chicken coleslaw 20
- Chickpea salad with zucchini and chilli 18
- Citrus fennel salad 18
- Fig and prosciutto salad with spiced quail 28
- Garden salad with avocado 22
- Pear and rocket salad 22
- Quinoa salad with mint and lemon 25
- Sweet potato, prosciutto and green bean salad 26

salsa
- Fresh tomato salsa 115
- Mango and cucumber salsa 32

San choi bow 82

sauces
- allergens in 10
- Caramel sauce 132, 140
- Chilli caramel sauce 42
- Chunky tomato and olive sauce 62
- Plum sauce 70
- Roast capsicum and tomato sauce 88
- Sage 'butter' sauce 42

sausages
- Curried sausage casserole 112

scones
- Date scones 152

Self-saucing banana pudding with caramel sauce 140

sesame seeds and their products 2, 4, 5

shellfish and their
  products 2, 3, 4, 5, 8

Smoked chicken pasta 36

smoothies
  Banana breakfast smoothie 14

snacks, allergens in 9

soups
  Chicken and corn soup 40
  Hearty vegetable soup 94
  Lamb shank and
    vegetable soup 54
  Lentil soup 94
  Pea and ham soup 67
  Thai pumpkin soup 96

soy beans and their
  products 4, 5, 6

spinach
  Curried spinach and
    capsicum kasha 98
  Spinach and
    capsicum muffins 14
  Spinach, pumpkin and
    sage polenta slice 92

Spring rolls 82

stew
  Lamb and vegetable stew 121

stir-fry
  Garlic pepper lamb stir-fry 72

sulphite preservatives 5

Sweet potato, prosciutto
  and green bean salad 26

tapioca flour 6

tarts
  Jamaican apple tart 136

Thai pumpkin soup 96

tomatoes
  Bacon and tomato
    stuffed mushrooms 15
  Chunky tomato
    and olive sauce 62
  Fresh tomato salsa 115
  Ratatouille 90
  Roast capsicum
    and tomato sauce 88
  Tomato relish 108

tree nuts and their
  products 2, 3, 4, 5

Vanilla frosting 160

veal
  Meatloaf with
    tomato relish 108
  Osso buco 74
  Veal with chunky tomato
    and olive sauce 62

vegetables
  allergens in 8
  Hearty vegetable soup 94
  Lamb shank and
    vegetable soup 54
  Lamb and vegetable stew 121
  see also specific vegetables

vegetarian products
  containing allergens 9

wheat products
  alternatives to 6
  allergy to 4, 5

zucchini
  Chickpea salad with
    zucchini and chilli 18
  Ratatouille 90

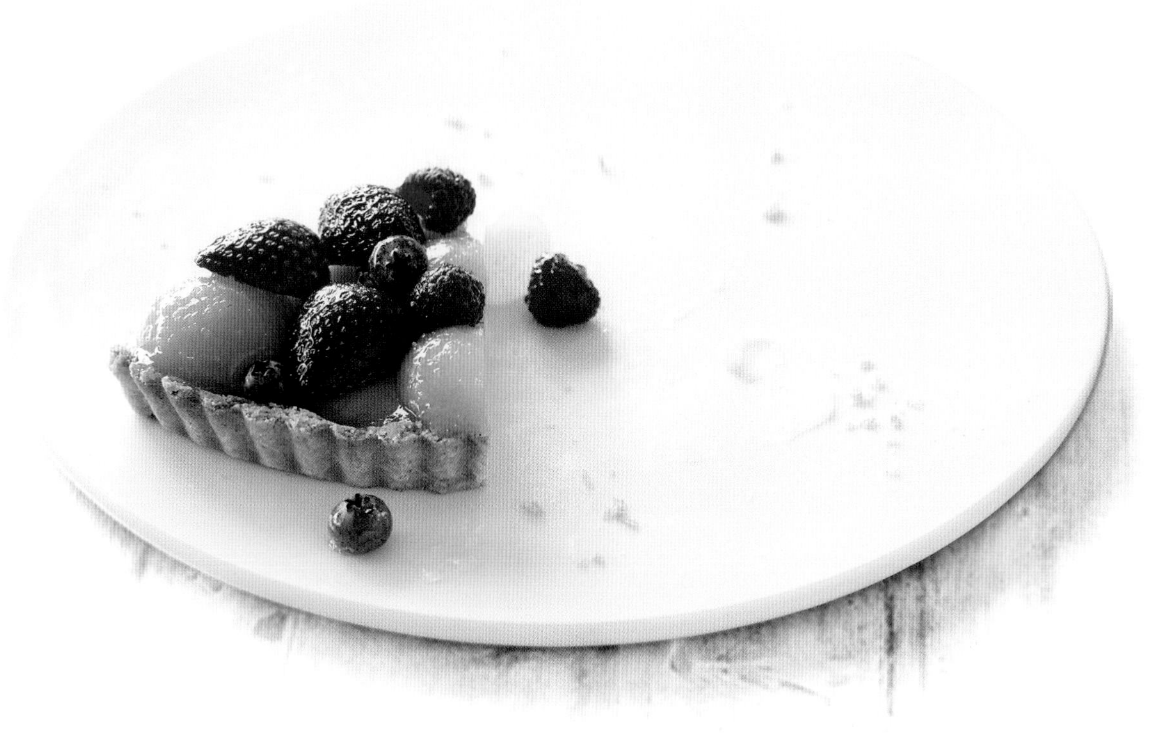

VIKING

Published by the Penguin Group
Penguin Group (Australia)
250 Camberwell Road, Camberwell, Victoria 3124, Australia
(a division of Pearson Australia Group Pty Ltd)
Penguin Group (USA) Inc.
375 Hudson Street, New York, New York 10014, USA
Penguin Group (Canada)
90 Eglinton Avenue East, Suite 700, Toronto, Canada ON M4P 2Y3
(a division of Pearson Penguin Canada Inc.)
Penguin Books Ltd
80 Strand, London WC2R 0RL, England
Penguin Ireland
25 St Stephen's Green, Dublin 2, Ireland
(a division of Penguin Books Ltd)
Penguin Books India Pvt Ltd
11 Community Centre, Panchsheel Park, New Delhi – 110 017, India
Penguin Group (NZ)
67 Apollo Drive, Rosedale, North Shore 0632, New Zealand
(a division of Pearson New Zealand Ltd)
Penguin Books (South Africa) (Pty) Ltd
24 Sturdee Avenue, Rosebank, Johannesburg 2196, South Africa

Penguin Books Ltd, Registered Offices:
80 Strand, London WC2R 0RL, England

First published by Penguin Group (Australia), 2012

10 9 8 7 6 5 4 3 2 1

Design by Ricardo Felipe © Penguin Group (Australia)
Photography by Rob Palmer
Styling by Michelle Noerianto
Typeset in Neuzeit 9.5/12.5pt by Post Pre-press Group, Brisbane, Queensland
Colour reproduction by Splitting Image Colour Studio Pty Ltd, Clayton, Victoria
Printed in China by South China Printing Co. Ltd.

National Library of Australia
Cataloguing-in-Publication data:
Shepherd, Sue.
Allergy-free cooking / Sue Shepherd.
9780670075539 (pbk.)
Includes index.
Food allergy – Diet therapy – Recipes.
Cooking.
641.56318

penguin.com.au

Front cover and previous page: Fruit custard flan, p 139
Back cover: Beef burritos, p 111